WORKSHOPS IN
BILE ACID RESEARCH

WORKSHOPS IN
BILE ACID RESEARCH

Serum Bile Acids in Health and Disease
and
The Pathophysiology of the Enterohepatic Circulation

From the 7th International Symposium on Bile Acids
held in Cortina D'Ampezzo, Italy, 17–20 March 1982

edited by

L. Barbara, R. H. Dowling,

A. Hofmann and E. Roda

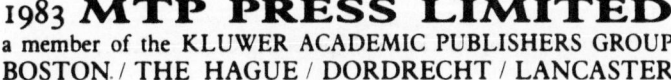
1983 **MTP PRESS LIMITED**
a member of the KLUWER ACADEMIC PUBLISHERS GROUP
BOSTON / THE HAGUE / DORDRECHT / LANCASTER

Published in the UK and Europe by
MTP Press Limited
Falcon House
Lancaster, England

British Library Cataloguing in Publication Data

Workshops in bile acid research.
1. Bile acids—Congresses
I. Barbara, L.
612'.35   QP 752.B54

ISBN-13:978-94-009-6618-5

Published in the USA by
MTP Press
A division of Kluwer Boston Inc
190 Old Derby Street
Hingham, MA02043, USA

Library of Congress Cataloging in Publication Data

Main entry under title:

Workshops in bile acid research.

Bibliography: p.
Includes index.
1. Liver—Diseases—Diagnosis—Congresses.
2. Bile acids—Diagnostic use—Congresses. 3. Bile
acids—Analysis—Congresses.   I. Barbara, L. (Luigi)
[DNLM: 1. Bile acids and salts—Congresses.
2. Bile acids and salts—Blood—Congresses. WI 703
B5953 1982]
RC847.B54 1983   616.3'6207576   83-17553
ISBN-13:978-94-009-6618-5   e-ISBN-13:978-94-009-6616-1
DOI: 10.1007/978-94-009-6616-1

Phototypeset by Blackpool Typesetting Services Ltd.,

Contents

Preface

During the 7th International Bile Acid meeting held in Cortina d'Ampezzo, Italy, during March 1982, there were two important Workshops dealing with recent advances in two areas of bile acid metabolism – Serum Bile Acids in Health and Disease and The Pathophysiology of the Enterohepatic Circulation. These Workshops complemented the broad range of topics in bile acid metabolism which were presented formally as part of a Postgraduate Course. The proceedings of these formal presentations have already been published by MTP Press under the title *Bile Acids in Gastroenterology* but in view of the exciting, important, new information which emerged during both Workshops, the organisers of the meeting felt that it would be valuable to record and edit the proceedings of the Workshops, which form the basis of this volume.

The advent of new techniques for measurement of total and individual bile acids in serum now means that accurate and reliable measurements of bile acids in peripheral circulation are available to all. This has resulted in a veritable explosion of information in the serum bile acid field and, therefore, the appearance of a critical evaluation of the technical and basic scientific and clinical aspects of measuring serum bile acids is indeed timely.

Partly as a result of these technical innovations there have also been interesting advances in our understanding of the enterohepatic circulation of bile acids and how this is disturbed in liver and intestinal disease. It is hoped that the Proceedings of these two Workshops will be of interest to basic scientists and clinical investigators alike.

The Editors are grateful to Dr Gian Germano Guiliani, Gipharmex SpA, Milan, whose generous support made the meeting possible, and also wish to thank Mr M. Lister, Managing Editor of MTP Press Limited, and Mrs Veronica Cesari, Italian Society of Gastroenterology, for their valuable help in the preparation of these Proceedings.

The Editors

SERUM BILE ACIDS
IN HEALTH AND DISEASE

Barbara: On behalf of my co-chairman, Dr Paumgartner from Münich, all my staff and of course myself, I welcome all the participants to this workshop.

The first part of the workshop, after a discussion of the current methodology, is dedicated to the study of the physiological mechanisms which influence and determine serum bile acid concentrations. Therefore the main determinants of serum bile acid levels in fasting and postprandial states will be discussed: for example, gastric emptying, gallbladder and biliary tract emptying and filling, intestinal motility and absorption, hepatic blood flow, hepatic uptake and transport.

The second part deals with the evaluation of serum bile acids in diagnosis.

The theme of the workshop has created some perplexity, largely because, up to this moment, there has not been enough clinical experience of such a diagnostic test. You may be surprised that we are proposing a new biochemical procedure, in a period in which traditional liver function tests are outmoded, and new diagnostic techniques are widely applied. However, we hold that this workshop is opportune because, for some time, the test has been adopted as standard practice in hospitals in Italy and elsewhere. The main prerequisites that we expect from a new biochemical test, without going into detail, are its specificity, sensitivity and predictive values.

So we need to answer some questions. Can the serum bile acids accurately discriminate between health and disease? Are they capable of distinguishing between various hepatobiliary diseases? If so, are they more useful than traditional liver function tests? Do serum bile acid tests add to our existing store of knowledge or are they an effective substitute for previous procedures?

I hope that this workshop will clarify some, if not all, of these points.

PART I

Paumgartner: In the first part of this workshop we shall discuss a few new important trends in methodology, and we shall then talk about the determinants of serum bile acids in health. As you all know, we can measure serum bile acids by enzymatic techniques, by immunoassays, by gas–liquid chromatography, either with packed columns or with capillary columns; finally, we can measure bile acids by capillary gas–liquid chromatography–mass spectrometry. These methods do not all measure the same bile acid species in serum. Their specificities and their sensitivities are different. Therefore for each purpose the optimal technique must be selected.

A problem that has been with us for quite some time, but that has never received sufficient attention, is the determination of the percentage of unconjugated bile acids in serum. This is probably due to methodological difficulties.

Dr Setchell will now tell us about his technique concerning the separation of unconjugated from conjugated serum bile acids.

Setchell: I described to you earlier two chromatographic techniques which are ideally suited to the separation and isolation of unconjugated bile acids in serum. The first technique involves the application of reverse phase octadecylsilane bonded silica in cartridges (Bond-

Elut). As I explained, this is a solid adsorbant which will extract, from aqueous solution, highly polar and medium-polarity lipophilic or amphiphic molecules. It can therefore be used for the extraction of unconjugated bile acids from serum samples, as well as all of the more polar conjugated bile acids (Setchell and Worthington, 1982). In addition it is a very useful method for de-salting the serum sample and for the removal of proteins and non-polar lipids, of which cholesterol is the major non-polar lipid in serum.

This extraction procedure affords an extract containing total bile acids. If we combine this technique with the use of the lipophilic gel, Lipidex 1000 (Fig. 1), which behaves in a contrasting manner to the Bond-Elut cartridge – that is by excluding polar compounds but adsorbing non-polar lipids from acidified aqueous solution – unconjugated bile acids will be quantitatively adsorbed to the lipophilic gel (Dyfverman and Sjövall, 1978).

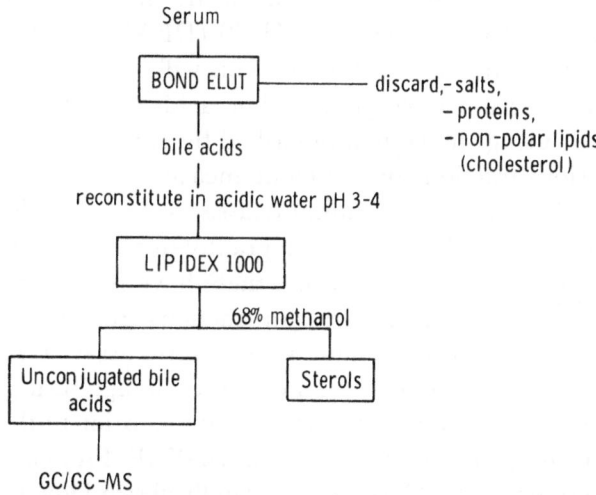

Figure 1 Capillary column gas chromatographic (GC) analysis of the methyl ester–trimethyl ether derivatives of serum bile acids in a sample from a fasting patient with an ileal resection. GC was carried out using a 25 m Silicone OV-1 glass capillary column and temperature programmed operation, 225–285 °C at 2 °C/min. (MS = mass spectrometry.)

With the use of a reverse phase solvent system, in this case 68% methanol, unconjugated bile acids can be recovered from the Lipidex 1000 and at the same time the small percentage of monohydroxy sterols that may still be present following the initial extracting will be retained by the gel (Setchell and Matsui, 1983).

Unconjugated bile acids can then be analysed by gas chromatography, or gas chromatography–mass spectrometry following the preparation of suitable derivatives.

There is one point I would like to stress about this technique: if any other method of detection is used, such as a radioimmunoassay or an enzyme method that will detect or has the capability of measuring glycine-conjugated bile acids then the chromatographic/isolation system is unsuitable. This is because – as I showed earlier – a small but variable proportion of glycine-conjugated bile acids are adsorbed from the acidic aqueous solution by Lipidex 1000, and these will interfere with the measurement of unconjugated bile acids.

This problem can be overcome by using an alternative method for isolating unconjugated bile acids. Thus having carried out the initial extraction stage with reverse phase octadecylsilane bonded silica cartridges, the extract containing total bile acids can be subjected to anion exchange chromatography using the lipophilic gel, diethylaminohydroxypropyl Sephadex LH 20 (DEAP-LH-20) or as it is commercially sold, Lipidex-DEAP. This will provide a very specific separation of serum unconjugated bile acids from those which are conjugated, using the system described by Almé et al., 1977.

The various fractions may then be measured using an enzymatic fluorometric assay or radioimmunoassay or, as we do, with gas chromatography and gas chromatography–mass spectrometry.

It has come to my attention that there have been some problems in the measurement of bile acids in fractions from Lipidex-DEAP, particularly when an enzymatic fluorometric assay is used. In the original method by Almé et al., a cation exchange resin, Amberlyst A-15, was used to remove interfering cations prior to the anion exchange chromatography step on Lipidex-DEAP. From data obtained in conjunction with Dr Gerry Murphy in Professor Dowling's department we have found that when this method is used the results that one obtained by enzyme fluorometry for the bile acid concentration in each of the conjugate fractions bore no relationship to the amount that one obtained if the serum sample was measured directly for total bile acids without this fractionation.

The problem of interference arises from the use of Amberlyst A-15. Those who may have used the Almé method with an enzyme fluorometric technique will obtain unfavourable results as a result of using Amberlyst A-15; however this problem may be satisfactorily overcome by substituting the cation exchange gel SP-Sephadex at this stage.

Figure 2 shows a capillary column gas chromatographic profile that is typical of the unconjugated bile acids in the fasting serum sample of a patient with an ileal resection. With this example I would like to rectify the misconception that gas chromatography–mass spec-'trometry is a non-sensitive technique, by carrying out some calculations based on this particular example.

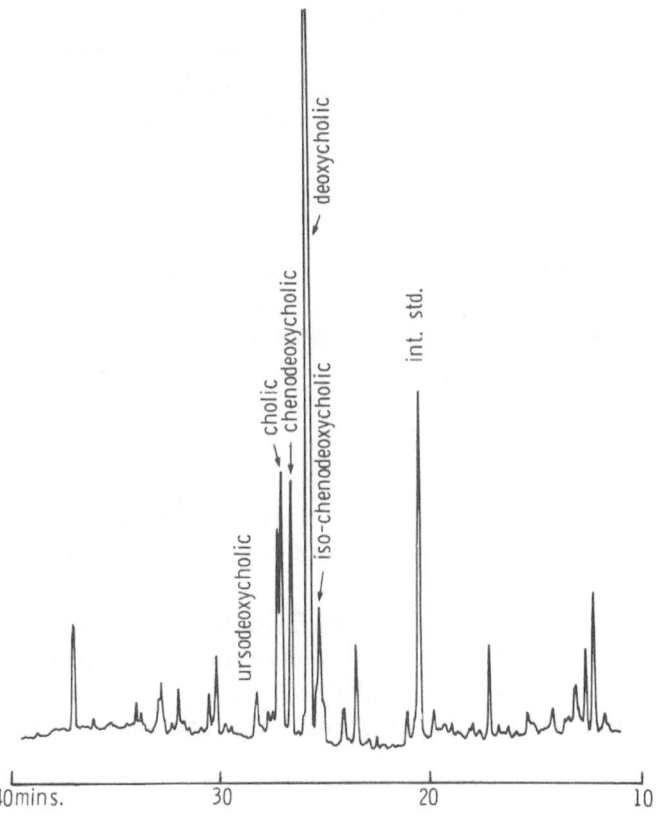

Figure 2   Capillary column gas chromatographic profile (see Text)

A full-scale deflection (FSD) for a peak on this chromatogram is obtained from approximately 50 ng of bile acid injected onto the column, and in this example one-twentieth of the total serum extract was injected. By my calculations the total amount of bile acid due to the peak for deoxycholic acid, will be 1000 ng. Assuming a molecular weight of approximately 400, we therefore have approximately 2.5 nmol of bile acid detected. Since this was from 2 ml of serum, a peak giving a full-scale deflection will arise from a bile acid with a concentration of 1 μmol/l, in serum.

We can, of course, quite easily measure peaks of 10% of that size, which thus gives a sensitivity, at 0.1 μmol/l, and furthermore since it is possible to inject up to half of the sample the limit of detection will be about 0.01 μmol/l and I think that probably compares fairly favourably with other immunoassay techniques. Perhaps somebody will correct me if I'm wrong.

Using this technique for unconjugated serum bile acids one can detect a number of different bile acids in the serum of patients with ileal resection and these were identified by gas chromatography–mass spectrometry. Recent work from our laboratory, and in collaboration with Dr G. Murphy, has revealed that unconjugated serum bile acids show a diurnal variation in healthy subjects, and these techniques are currently being used for similar studies in patients with ileal resections (Setchell, *et al.*, 1982).

An alternative to gas chromatography is to utilize gas chromatography–mass spectrometry for the measurement of bile acids in the unconjugated fraction. By using the technique of selected ion monitoring it is possible to select ions which are characteristic of monohydroxy, dihydroxy and trihydroxy bile acids, and by simultaneously monitoring the gas chromatographic effluent, it is possible to detect with high sensitivity bile acids with these general structures.

I think probably I should just finish by saying that the sensitivity of gas chromatography–mass spectrometry is approximately 100-fold greater than that of capillary column gas chromatography, which means that we should have a sensitivity of between 0.001 and 0.0001 μmol/l.

Paumgartner: Even after group separation, as Dr Setchell said, and even using capillary gas–liquid chromatography, specific and sensitive measurement, especially of minor species of bile acids in serum, may be difficult.

Dr Stellaard will describe some data which illustrate this methodological difficulty and the advantages of mass spectrometry, and then there will be a discussion of these two things and the presentation of Dr Roda together, because these deal with mass spectrometry to a certain extent, so I would like to ask Dr Stellaard to show his data very briefly.

Stellaard: I would like to present some preliminary data from our laboratory on the use of capillary gas chromatography–mass spectrometry for the detection of bile acids in health.

As Dr Setchell pointed out, even after careful sample preparation and the use of capillary gas chromatography (GC), many peaks may remain unresolved. We support, therefore, the idea that it is necessary to measure serum bile acids with the highest specificity possible: that is capillary GC in combination with mass spectrometry (MS).

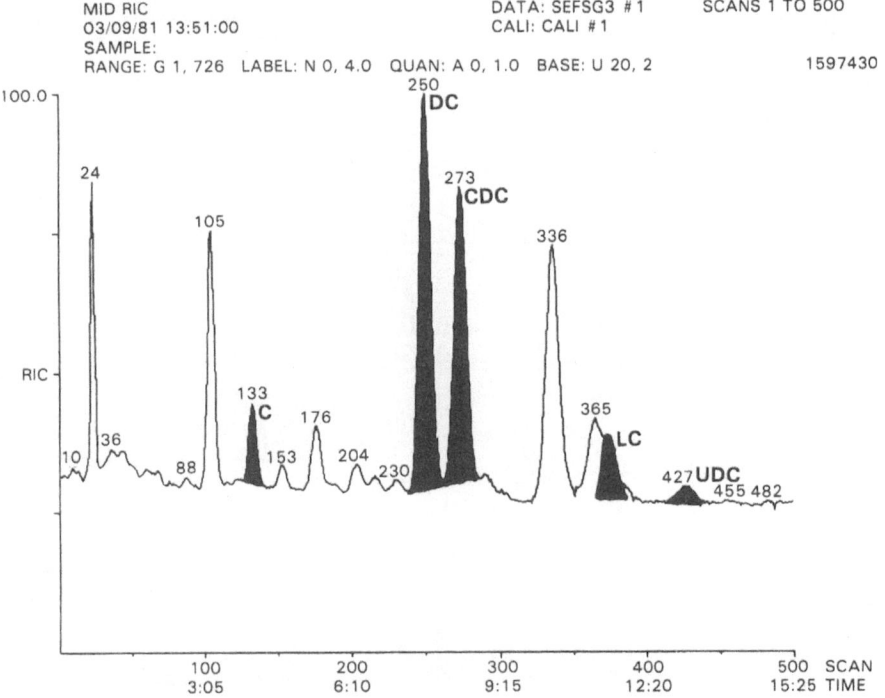

Figure 3 Total line chromatogram after a capillary GC/MS run of a serum sample from a healthy person. C = cholic acid; DC = deoxycholic acid; CDC = chenodeoxycholic acid; LC = lithocholic acid; UDC = ursodeoxycholic acid

Figure 3 shows a total line chromatogram after a capillary GC/MS run of a serum sample of a healthy person. This chromatogram is, in principle, comparable to a tracing you will obtain running GC with a flame ionization detection. You see the peaks as they are indicated. The cholic acid peak, deoxycholic acid peak, cheno and urso.

Now I would like to focus on the lithocholic acid peak, and it is quite obvious that this peak is overlapping with other peaks, eluting around the same retention time, and with GC only, quantitation and detection of lithocholic acid will be in danger. Therefore it needs mass spectrometry with an adequate data system to acquire complete separation, as shown in Fig. 4.

On the bottom you see the same tracing as in Fig. 3. The tracings above are so-called mass chromatograms, as Dr Setchell showed in a somewhat different way, showing the same compounds but in their specific ions, and we see that in specific ion 372, the lithocholic acid has been completely separated from anything else eluting at the time point.

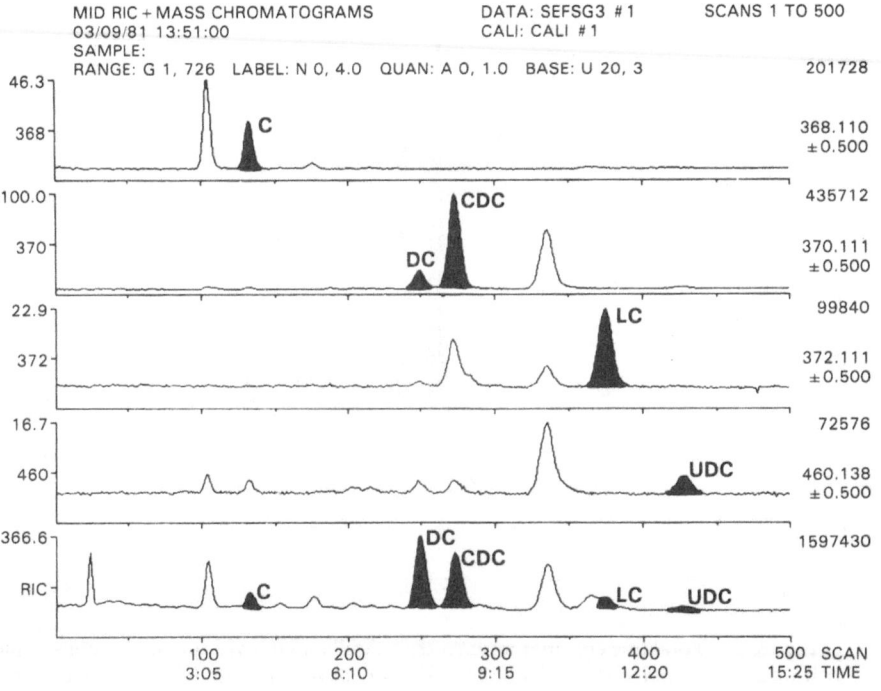

Figure 4

The high specificity of MS also permits the detection of minor species of bile acid in serum, even of healthy subjects. Table 1 shows you the results obtained in a five-fold determination on a pool containing postprandial serum of a group of healthy subjects. At first, when we look at the different types of bile acids, we see the normal ones that we expect. In addition, we find a couple of others, including hyocholic acid, the 3-beta-delta-5, that many people have already been looking for in normal serum and two iso bile acids from deoxy and cheno.

Then I would like to point out the accuracy of measurement when we look at the reproducibility over five determinations. With the exception of one the reproducibility is better than 10%. In this range, of the iso bile acids, we are looking at about 2%, between 1 and 2% of the total bile acid concentration present in the sample.

Table 1

	Concentration (μmol/l)	C.V. (%)
Cholic acid	0.42 ± 0.03	6.0
Deoxycholic acid	1.36 ± 0.06	4.3
Chenodeoxycholic acid	1.49 ± 0.05	3.1
Lithocholic acid	0.47 ± 0.03	7.3
Ursodeoxycholic acid	0.30 ± 0.01	4.5
Hyocholic acid	0.19 ± 0.01	4.7
3β-5-Cholenoic acid	0.34 ± 0.01	2.6
Isodeoxycholic acid	0.12 ± 0.01	11.2
Isochenodeoxycholic acid	0.11 ± 0.05	4.1
Total	4.80 ± 0.17	3.6

Stellaard: I would like to make one statement and to provide one illustration. It should be pointed out that with MS also the separation of the ^{12}C and ^{13}C contributions in a compound can be accomplished, allowing isotope ratio measurements. This makes it possible to measure stable isotope-labelled bile acids in serum after oral or intravenous administration of 24-^{13}C-labelled bile acids.

As pointed out by Dr Hofmann, this permits the measurements of bile acid kinetics by non-invasive techniques.

To demonstrate the technical ability of making those measurements, Figure 5 shows the atom per cent excess value expressing the excess ^{13}C label present in the substance, measured in serum for cheno, lithocholic and ursodeoxycholic acid. This is a kind of demonstration where you can see that the label of chenodeoxycholic acid disappears from cheno and appears in the lithocholic and ursodeoxycholic acid. That has been done after administration of 50 mg of 24-^{13}C chenodeoxycholic acid.

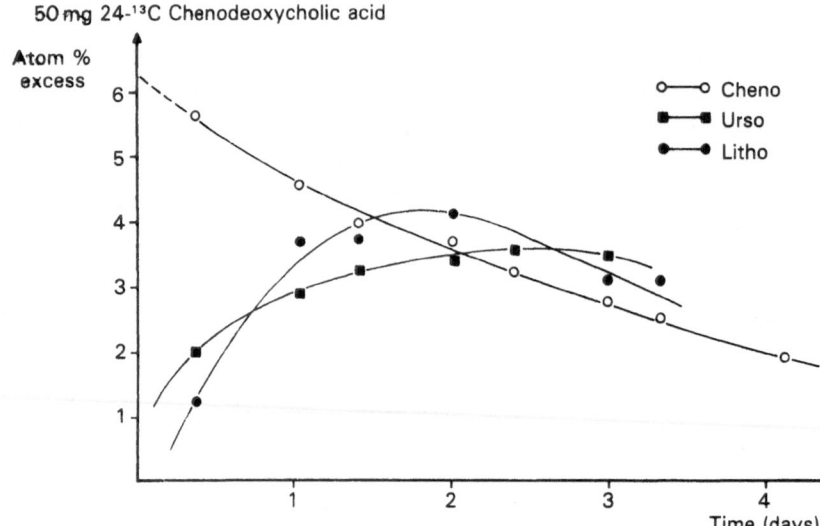

Figure 5

Paumgartner: Now after Dr Stellaard has shown you how things can become difficult and complex when you want to measure a wide spectrum of bile acids, Dr Aldo Roda will show you how the primary bile acids in serum, which possess a 7-alpha hydroxy group, can be measured very rapidly with a fascinating new technique which he has developed very recently.

Roda: In order to measure the serum primary bile acids with adequate sensitivity, we developed a new highly sensitive enzymatic bio-luminescent assay. The method is basically based on the use of three enzymes: 7-alpha-hydroxysteroid dehydrogenase (7-alpha-HSD), NADH-FMN oxidoreductase (NADH-FMN ox-rd), and bacterial luciferase. The principle of the method is as follows: the 7-alpha-HSD catalyses the oxidation of the 7-alpha-hydroxyl of the bile acid to 7-keto group. The NADH formed is utilized by the second enzyme, i.e. NADH-FMN ox-rd that converts FMN in its reduced form. The third enzyme, i.e. luciferase using $FMNH_2$ and decanal, catalyses the production of light. The peak intensity of the emitted light is proportional to the amount of bile acid present in the sample.

From the analytical point of view the method is very rapid, no incubation time is required. The three enzymes are immobilized and so rinsable. The signal is stable for at least 2–3 min. The light is recorded by a relatively simple and inexpensive instrument such as a luminometer. The sensitivity of the method is high, i.e. 1 pmol/tube comparable to that of immunological methods. In addition the method is highly specific for 2-alpha-hydroxy bile acid, and other steroids present in serum do not interfere. There is a good correlation with other independent methods such as gas–liquid chromatography (GLC) and radioimmunoassay (RIA). This method appears a valid alternative to the conventional methods for bile acids thanks to its extremely high sensitivity and precision, and to the relatively low cost.

Paumgartner: Now questions to Dr Setchell, Dr Stellaard and Dr Roda.

Roda: I have a question for Dr Setchell in terms of sensitivity of the method. You report a sensitivity for GC of $0.01\,\mu mol/l$, but how many ml? What is the volume of the starting sample?

Setchell: That particular example was 2 ml of serum but in most circumstances we analyse around 1 ml of serum. I think you have to bear in mind that we are injecting on the instrument the equivalent of only $20\,\mu l$ of serum (i.e. one-fiftieth of total extract) and that is important because, in fact, the technique renders itself very useful for the analysis of samples from newborn infants.

Unidentified Discussant: Dr Setchell. The bile acid concentrations you have shown us in patient with ileal resection, were these unconjugated bile acids?

Setchell: They were only unconjugated bile acids.

Hofmann: It seems to me that the reason we cannot separate the glycine conjugates from the unconjugated bile acids by simple absorption techniques is because the glycine makes the bile acids more polar and therefore when we have glycine-conjugated, mono-hydroxy bile acids, they are similar in polarity to unconjugated tri-hydroxy bile acids. We solve this problem by taking advantage of the different strengths of the acidity of the glycine by using a weak anion exchange column. So my question is this: is it permissible to take the fraction containing the mixture of glycine conjugates and unconjugates and put it directly onto the GC and let the GC graph do the sorting for you, because all that will come out in the GC is the unconjugated bile acids?

Setchell: Yes, you can do that. Regarding your first point: I think the reason that Lipidex 1000 adsorbs glycine conjugates is more likely to be due to some ion pair effect which is variable and depends upon the type of sample. It is not entirely a polarity effect, but perhaps an ion pair effect. You are quite correct in your second point. Even if glycine conjugated bile acids are present in the final extract for GC–MS analysis, they will not be eluted from the GC column, or more correctly will take many hours to elute, so they will, in fact, not interfere with the unconjugated bile acid methyl ester–trimethylsilyl ethers.

Dowling: I would like to ask all three speakers, but perhaps Dr Stellaard in particular, about the problem that we have often had; that is, a discrepancy between the serum total bile acid measurement, as calculated, for example, by an enzymatic fluorometric assay, and the summation of the individual bile acids as demonstrated by RIA or GC–MS or capillary chromatography. Because there is often a gap between the two, it seems to me that with increasing sensitivity we are detecting many more minor bile acids, but the conventional major four bile acids in the serum and in bile are not adequate to account for the total that we can measure by an enzymatic assay. Is there still a gap by the summation of the individual bile acids with these methods?

Stellaard: The data that I showed on Fig. 5 were as follows: the 3-beta substance that we found calculated for about 10% of the total concentration. So that would not be a great factor in the differences that one sees comparing the methods.

Dowling: I think the problem is not so much 3-beta. Obviously with an enzymatic fluorometric assay you can either choose to use a 3-alpha or beta or both, and you end up with a total. The question is: if you take all your individual bile acids and sum them, is there still a difference from the total as measured by an enzymatic fluorometric assay which will record both alpha and beta configuration bile acids?

Stellaard: We did not yet make comparison studies between enzymatic methods and GC–MS, but I can say already, and maybe Dr Setchell has data on it, that when we compared GC with GC–MS we get really large differences.

Paumgartner: It could be helpful to give the means of bile acids which one finds by the various methods in fasting normal subjects. With the 3-alpha hydroxy-steroid dehydrogenase method we get a normal mean of $4.6 \pm 2.9\,\mu$mol/l. If we use capillary GLC we get $2.1 \pm 1.2\,\mu$mol/l. This difference can be explained by a certain unspecificity of the enzymatic method. If we use RIA, namely the kit from Becton Dickinson, which mainly measures conjugated cholate and conjugated chenodeoxycholate, we get a mean of $1.7 \pm 1.0\,\mu$mol/l in the same group of healthy subjects. If you compare these measurements, the enzymatic method gives the highest values followed by GLC and RIA.

Setchell: I think the answer is relatively simple and that is really that you cannot compare the two types of techniques. I think that one would expect perhaps the physical techniques of measurement, i.e. GC or more specifically GC–MS, to give much lower values than the relatively non-specific techniques. In my opinion if one tries to 'cut corners' by reducing the time of analysis then inevitably something has to suffer, and I think that the result is an assay which is less specific and subject to greater interference. This is really the simple answer to the differences that one gets between the two techniques.

Some recent work from Dr Murphy's laboratory showed that when bile acids were measured in samples by an enzymatic fluorometric method after they had been fractionated on Lipidex-DEAP according to the method described by Almé et al. (1977), the sum of the values for each conjugate group was many times greater than the value obtained when the serum was assayed without the fractionation step. Investigations of the method revealed that gross interference arose from the use of Amberlyst A-15 resin in the method. However, when this cation exchanger was replaced with the cation exchange gel SP-Sephadex no interference occurred, and the sum of the values for the bile acid concentration in each fraction approximated that for the total concentration in the serum assayed directly. This is an excellent example of interference or non-specificity in an assay system.

Roda: I just want to add one point about the enzymatic method using a 3-alpha-hydroxy steroid hydrogenase. We normally have an over-estimation when we measure bile acids with this method for one reason: some commercial available dehydrogenases are not completely specific for acidic steroids such as BA. For example a 3-alpha-HSD from Sigma catalyses also the oxidation of the alpha-hydroxy sterols. The amount of serum needed for BA analysis is in the order of 0.5–2 ml and even if the other steroids are present in the serum at a concentration ten times less than that of BA, a possible interference (over-estimation) might occur.

Paumgartner: Thank you very much. There is no question that the enzymatic method is the least specific and gives the highest values.

Fromm: A very short question to Dr Stellaard. I noticed that in your list of bile acids identified in the serum, you did not list 7-ketolithocholic acid and especially not in your description of the bile transformation of chenodeoxycholic acid to ursodeoxycholic acid.

Stellaard: Not at all.

Paumgartner: We shall now go on to another important topic of this workshop and I should like to start the discussion of some of the determinants of serum bile acid (SBA) concentrations in health. We are going to discuss disease in the second part of this workshop.

The concentrations of bile acids in serum are determined by the instantaneous balance between intestinal absorption of bile acids and hepatic elimination of bile acids. In the first part of this discussion we shall talk about the factors influencing intestinal input of bile acids. I should like to ask Dr Festi to tell us something about the delivery of bile acids into the duodenum in the fasting state and after meals and the correlation of this delivery of bile acids into the duodenum with SBA levels.

Festi: As far as the fasting state is concerned, we have evaluated gall-bladder motility and SBA levels in one normal subject during an overnight fast. Gallbladder emptying was evaluated by ultrasound and SBA concentrations by RIA. After the emptying induced by the evening meal, the gallbladder remained contracted until the early morning, when its refilling occurred, although interrupted by some spontaneous contractions (15–20% of reduction in volume). SBA levels increased after gallbladder emptying, returning to baseline during fasting.

In order to define the role of gallbladder motility as a determinant of SBA levels, we performed a study aimed to correlate gallbladder emptying, induced by both a standard solid meal (1000 cal.) and a cerulein infusion $(2 \, ng \, (kg \, bw)^{-1} \, min^{-1} \times 5 \, min)$ to SBA levels.

We have studied 40 subjects: 20 normal subjects, 10 with functioning (N) and 10 with sluggish gallbladder (NP), 10 cholesterol gallstone patients (GP) with functioning gallbladder and 10 cholecystectomized patients (C).

SBA levels were measured by specific RIA and the results expressed as area under the curve (AUC/180 min). Biliary tract emptying was evaluated using a cholescintigraphic technique (^{99m}Tc HIDA).

SBA levels after both cerulein and meal administration displayed a biphasic behaviour in N, NP and GP, with an early peak (within 30 min) and a second peak after 90 min. The first peak increased progressively from N to GP and NP (20, 30 and 45% of the total AUC). In C a single peak was noted, which accounted for 65% of the total AUC. No correlation was found between the percentage of gallbladder emptying ($71.4 \pm 3.2\%$ in N, $31.7 \pm 8.0\%$ in NP and $48.8 \pm 3.9\%$ in GP) and SBA AUC.

The occurrence in all patients of an early peak, not related to biliary tract emptying, suggests the presence in the intestine of a fraction of the bile acid pool in the fasting state. To confirm this hypothesis we measured SBA levels in two normal subjects and two cholecystectomized patients after duodenal infusion of sorbitol, a substance known to stimulate intestinal, but not biliary tract, motility (Fig. 6). The lack of gallbladder contraction during sorbitol infusion was checked, in the two normal subjects, by ultrasound.

In both groups of subjects SBA increased during the infusion, supporting our hypothesis and suggesting also that the intestine plays and important role in defining the shape of SBA concentrations.

Paumgartner: Before discussing this paper it would be very interesting to ask Dr Roda about the effect of the composition of meals on gallbladder emptying and the relation of gallbladder emptying after meals to SBA levels. We could then discuss both presentations together.

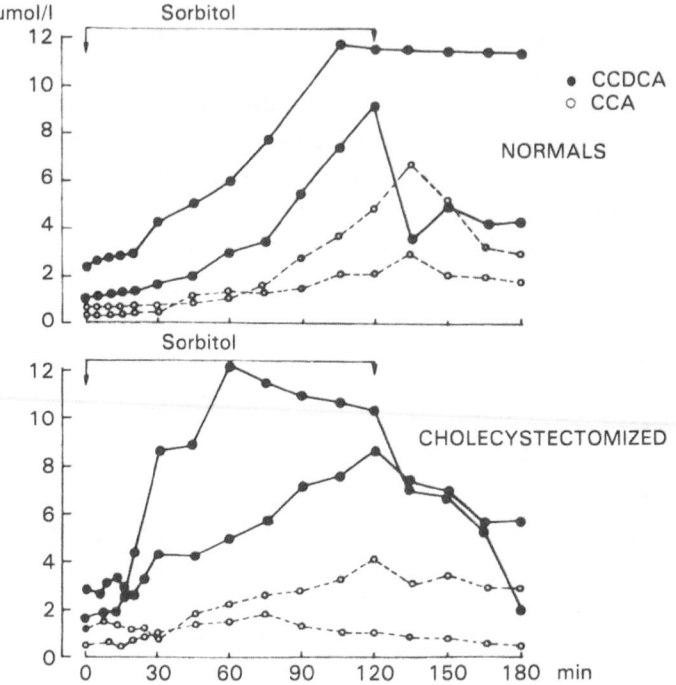

Figure 6   Serum bile acid levels in normal and cholecystectomized patients

Roda: The aim of our work was to evaluate the effect of varying meal weight and composition on gallbladder emptying and SBA levels. Five normal subjects were given two prefixed and equilibrated meals (A and C, Table 2) and a self-selected filling meal (B). Meal B was more rich in lipids than the others, but similar to meal C in weight and calories.

Table 2   Effect of varying meal weight and composition on gallbladder emptying and serum bile acid levels

Meal	A	B	C
Weight (g)	300	803 ± 150	900
Total caloric intake (kcal)	398	1103 ± 240	1194
Proteins (kcal)	107	229 ± 108	322
Fats (kcal)	36	383 ± 97	107
Carbohydrates (kcal)	255	516 ± 230	764
Liquid/solid ratio	1.0	1.3 ± 0.14	1.0
Gallbladder emptying (%)	39.7 ± 7.30	75.8 ± 6.92	43.5 ± 14.0
CCA AUC (μmol/l × 180 min)	0.62 ± 0.28	1.25 ± 0.54	2.43 ± 1.10
CCDCA AUC (μmol/l × 180 min)	1.70 ± 0.88	3.64 ± 1.37	4.40 ± 2.10

Gallbladder emptying was evaluated by an ultrasound technique and the results were expressed as percentage reduction of the initial volume; serum levels of cholic (CCA) and chenodeoxycholic (CCDCA) acid conjugates were measures by specific RIAs, and the results expressed as area under the curve/180 min. As far as gallbladder emptying was concerned, meal B induced a significantly greater emptying than meals A and C; no difference was observed between meal A and C. CCA and CCDCA AUC progressively increased from meal A to meal B and C, i.e. in relation to increasing weight and calories of the meal. We did not find any correlation between gall bladder emptying and SBA levels.

These preliminary data suggest that the meal composition, and particularly its lipid content, influences gallbladder emptying. The SBA AUC seems related mainly to the weight and calories of the meal.

Hofmann: I would like to congratulate the Bologna group on extending our knowledge in two ways. Firstly I think we have all known that part of the bile acid pool is in the intestine, but to date we have not done many experiments to learn about it and this is the first view that the fasting state content of the intestine is important in the SBA level, even in normal people. Secondly, I suggest that the work of La Russo (I will blame it on him seeing as it doesn't seem to be completely correct that in Rochester we missed part of an early peak in our cholecystectomized patients, because we didn't sample off enough). So it looks to me as if the postprandial rise in the cholecystectomized patient is more complicated than we thought, and I think that this is very interesting.

Paumgartner: Do you know to what extent unconjugated bile acids are responsible for this particular increase?

Setchell: Can I make one comment concerning the pool in the intestine? The pool in the intestine, particularly the large intestine, is most likely to be unconjugated, as you point out, and we find a postprandial increase in the serum unconjugated bile acids within 30 min of a meal. This obviously cannot be coming from gallbladder bile and probably reflects the fact that one has this bile acid pool sequestered in the intestinal lumen awaiting reabsorption.

Paumgartner: No, it is just that you said that this cannot possibly come from gallbladder contractions. But it could have some non-ionic passive absorption of the glycine conjugated cheno, for instance.

Setchell: I'm referring to the unconjugated bile acids, and of course, they are not present in bile in any significant quantities.

Unidentified Discussant: But glycine conjugates, cheno, would be in bile and could already start recirculating after 30 min. So you would also have a fraction of conjugated bile acids which could appear very early because they are absorbed in more proximal parts of the duodenum.

Corazziari: With regard to Dr Festi's presentation: if I recall correctly, he didn't see any gallbladder contraction during fasting. It is known that during the interdigestive period bile can be collected in the phase three period. So can he comment on whether this bile does not come from the gallbladder – or whether the methodology he uses is not sensitive enough to detect small gallbladder contractions.

Festi: We believe that ultrasonography represents a useful and reliable technique to study gallbladder emptying. Furthermore it allows the evaluation of gallbladder refilling. As far as the interdigestive migrating myoelectric complex is concerned, I have no data, but I suppose the gallbladder contracts spontaneously during the night in relation to the cyclical pattern of the interdigestive gastrointestinal motility.

Fromm: I think the immediate postprandial peak of unconjugated bile acids in serum can be explained by the gastrocholic reflex, because as soon as you get a meal into the stomach there is colonic motility. I think this would promote the reabsorption of unconjugated bile acids. I think that this is a very reasonable explanation.

Hofmann: I think the current view of intestinal motility between meals is that there is an interdigestive complex sweeping down the small intestine with a total small intestinal transit time of about 40 min. In principle, with the method of Dr Roda, we ought to be able to see the interdigestive complex producing an elevation in fasting bile acids every 40 min. If we do it will be very fascinating because we will have a non-invasive way of looking at the interdigestive complex. However, it is very bad, because those of us who work in bile acid will then have to go to motility meetings.

Paumgartner: Depending on the interdigestive complex, hepatic secretion of bile acids increases when the bile acids arrive in the ileum and are rapidly transported back to the liver. This has very nicely been shown by Peterson and co-workers.

Blum: The complex occurs every 90 min, not every 40.

Thistle: Although this has therapeutic implications, it is very much involved in our recent discussion, because saturation of bile is very dependent on the bile acid flux through the liver and bile becomes saturated in the early morning hours. It is apparent that if one could stimulate this bile acid flux through the liver beginning at 3, 4 or 5 a.m., one might have a very good way to prevent gallstones, and I wonder if some of the workers who are involved in gallbladder and small bowel motility and bile acid serum levels, considered this, and have any good approaches to, for example, delayed stimulations of the CCK.

Paumgartner: Now we shall have a pertinent contribution about intestinal motility. Dr Angelico will tell us something about the relation of bowel movements to serum bile acid levels.

Angelico: Within an epidemiological study on the prevalence of gallbladder disease in a female population of Rome (GREPCO), we have measured fasting primary serum bile acids (SBA), as a liver function test, using a commercially available radioimmunoassay (RIA). This preliminary report deals with the first 795 females so far examined.

During the study we employed a questionnaire to obtain some data and in each subject we also collected data on the frequency of bowel movements (Fig. 7). Excluding cholecystectomized subjects, we found that 18 females had habitually more than two evacuations per day; 551 females had one or two daily evacuations; 217 had one evacuation every 2 or 3 days, and 39 evacuated only less than once every 3 days.

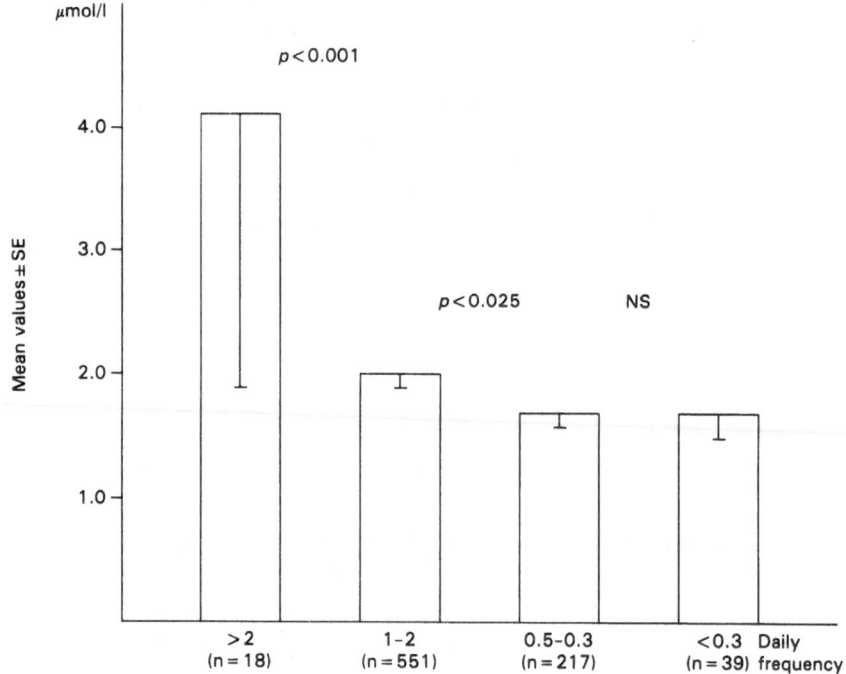

Figure 7 Fasting serum bile acids levels according to bowel frequency in 795 females (cholecystectomized subjects excluded)

The mean levels of primary SBA were significantly higher in the first group with respect to the others. The first group, however, is a small group with a high standard error. More interestingly, a statistical difference was observed also between the two major groups: in fact, females with one or two daily evacuations had significantly higher values of SBA than females who evacuated once every 2 or 3 days. At present we do not have an explanation for these findings, which, as mentioned, are related only to primary SBA. This observation might be changed measuring also the secondary bile acids in serum.

Hofmann: I would like to make a few brief comments about unconjugated bile acids in the intestine. First, as you all know, many bile acids come from the intestine. They are the primary conjugated bile acids, they are unconjugated bile acids, they are iso-bile acids and are cheto bile acids.

When they come to the liver they reach what you could consider to be the hepatic bile acid processing centre, and then the liver has to 'decide' what to do with all the strange bile acids. With Franz Stellaard we have studied the biliary bile acids in the National Gallstones Study by mass spectroscopy in the laboratory of Peter Klein, and there are only six main bile acids: the major primary and secondary bile acids, and a few patients have ursocholic. The reason is – in my opinion – that the liver is either bio-transforming to bile acids, for example, converting the iso-acids to 3-alpha, reducing the keto acids, the 3-keto, the 7-keto or the 12-keto and also conjugating the unconjugated acids. Other unusual exotic bile acids are rejected by the liver and they are eliminated in the urine, and therefore I think this is why we will find unusual bile acids in blood and the commoner bile acids in bile.

I would like to say two things about the unconjugated bile acids. First, as background, we know that the unconjugated bile acids are formed during digestion by bacteria in health and disease. This really derives from two kinds of experiments: bio-transformation experiments showing that if you give labelled taurocholate, the cholate moiety ends up in the glycine fraction; also work by Hans Fromm, who showed that the CO_2 is rapidly enriched if glycine is labelled in the carboxyl group.

We also know that unconjugated bile acids are rapidly and passively absorbed, and finally we know that the first-pass clearance of the unconjugated bile acids is relatively less. In other words, conjugated cheno might have 80% clearance, unconjugated might have 60% first-pass clearance, so that the peripheral levels are always enriched in unconjugated bile acids.

The rules, or the evidence, for the passive uptake, are mainly three. First, an extensive work by Dr Dietschy, who, unfortunately, could not be here, Dr Schiff and Dr Wilson, showing rapid passive uptake by duodenal segments. Perfusion studies with unconjugated chenodeoxycholate, by Gerard Van Berge-Henegouwen and also by Maurizio Ponz De Leon have shown that chenodeoxycholate is rapidly and passively absorbed in the duodenum, and then we have chronic feeding studies by people such as Dr LaRusso, who have fed deoxycholic, which suggested it is efficiently absorbed.

The view is that if, in a perfusion study, you plot concentration against the rate of absorption, you get a line, and its slope is in fact the permeability which is also approximately the same as the clearance.

The rules are, then, that the clearance of the unconjugated bile acids is directly proportional to the partition coefficient between octinol and water, and if one has this line of clearance the unconjugated bile acids are at the bottom, for example taurocholate. The less polar conjugates, such as the glycine dihydroxy bile acids, have the higher partition coefficient, some passive absorption and the unconjugated bile acids have rapid passive absorption.

Paumgartner: This is a good point now to move over to the second part of this discussion of physiological factors determining serum bile acids, namely to hepatic factors. Perhaps we could also discuss how important, in absolute terms, passive non-ionic uptake of bile acids by the liver is. As Dr Hofmann has shown, unconjugated bile acids will be taken up better by passive mechanisms than conjugated ones but, in absolute terms, this may not be important. I think that this is a point of uncertainty so far.

Let me now start the discussion of hepatic factors. Hepatic elimination of bile acids occurs during the first passage from portal blood and then, after their recirculation via the systemic circulation, both from portal and arterial blood.

Systemic clearance of the bile acids depends on the intrinsic clearance of bile acids and on liver blood flow. It is very important for our further discussion that the hepatic transport mechanisms responsible for bile acid uptake operate far below saturation both in normal subjects and also in patients with mild to moderate liver disease. Therefore the extraction fraction remains practically constant over the whole range of physiological bile acid loads to the liver. This should be kept in mind and this point should be considered in our further discussions of hepatic mechanisms regulating serum bile acid levels. Dr Aldini will start this part of the workshop showing her studies on bile acid uptake by the isolated perfused rat liver.

Aldini: The work that I am reporting concerns the effect of different parameters on the hepatic uptake of bile acids. We did single-pass rat liver perfusion experiments and equilibrium dialysis studies. We evaluated the effect of conjugation, number and position of hydroxyl groups and the effect of albumin binding on the hepatic uptake of bile acids. To evaluate the effect of conjugation we infused taurocholic acid, glycocholic acid and cholic acid. The hepatic uptake was higher for taurine conjugated that for glycine conjugated and for free cholic acid respectively. On the contrary, the relative percentage of albumin bound of the three bile acids (taurine and glycine conjugated and free form) was not significantly different (42%, 45% and 48% respectively at 3% albumin concentration).

As far as the number and the position of hydroxyl groups is concerned, cholic acid was taken up by the liver more efficiently that the two dihydroxy bile acids (chenodeoxycholic and ursodeoxycholic acids). The two dihydroxy bile acids were taken up more efficiently than the monohydroxy bile acid (lithocholic acid). 7-Ketolithocholic acid was taken up a little less than the trihydroxy bile acid, but more than the dihydroxy ones.

A third set of experiments was carried out with glycocholic acid, glycochenodeoxycholic acid and glycolithocholic acid at two different albumin concentrations in the medium (3 and 0.75%). This was at two different concentrations of bile acids: at tracer doses and at higher concentrations of bile acids (about $100 \mu mol/l$) that, in a final volume of 2.5 ml, gives about 25 nmol/g of liver. That is a dose fairly inferior to the one known to saturate the transport system.

When the albumin concentration in the medium was lowered from 3% to 0.75% the uptake of glycocholic acid at a tracer dose and, similarly, the extent of the albumin binding were decreased. But glycocheno- and glycolithocholates were taken up in a similar manner at the two concentrations and we did not find any difference in the albumin binding.

When we infused glycocholic acid and glycochenodeoxycholic acid at a dose of 25 nmol/g of liver, we found an increase in the uptake for both bile acids and similarly a decrease in the percentage of albumin binding.

In summary, the extent of albumin binding decreases from lithocholic acid to cholic acid, through chenodeoxycholic acid and ursodeoxycholic acid and it is inversely related to the hepatic extraction. A similar trend was observed for the hepatic extraction of glycoconjugated bile acids that parallels that of the free bile acids but was shifted to higher values of hepatic extraction. Therefore we can conclude that both differences in the moiety of the bile acids and differences in the albumin binding may be determinants of the hepatic bile acid uptake but the uptake of conjugated bile acids is also related to other factors such as interactions between albumin and the liver cell surface.

Paumgartner: In many points this fits very well studies which we have done together with Jütg Reichen in Berne, and it also fits observations of others in man, who have shown that taurocholate is taken up more efficiently by the liver than cholic acid. You have shown that taurocholate is taken up better than glycocholate and that a certain correlation exists between up-take rates and protein binding. That is very interesting.

Fromm: I have a question for Dr Aldini. Apparently from your presentation, I assume that serum albumin concentrations could very much modulate serum bile acids. Have you done any studies for some liver disease? I think we may not have thought at this point that since in liver disease the albumin concentration can vary, there are a number of patients with hypoalbuminaemia and many patients with normal albumin levels. Have you done any studies about this? Since we know that, for example, serum fasting levels and postprandial levels frequently are normal in patients with liver disease, have you studied serum albumin as a modulator of serum bile acids from this point of view?

Aldini: No, we have not any data about different serum albumin concentrations in humans. We have performed only liver perfusion experiments and *in vitro* studies to evaluate the possible role of albumin concentrations and bile acid–albumin binding on the bile acid liver uptake, but we have not any data on humans.

Paumgartner: It would be very interesting to perform studies similar to those of Rudy Schmidt with BSP in patients with nephrotic syndrome and very low serum albumin. It should be studied whether manipulation of serum albumin in these given patients influences the serum bile acid levels and bile acid clearance.

Fromm: We did this in some patients with nephrotic syndrome and we measured the serum bile acid concentration and, in fact, they are very low. The impression is that in chronic liver failure (just an impression), there is not so much correlation between the serum bile acid levels and albumin; furthermore I wonder whether, carrying on this type of study in human patients, it will be easy to distinguish between cause and effect.

Hofmann: In the past our group has looked at the effect of albumin concentration. My personal belief is that the changes which occur in liver disease will not be important in bile acid binding. What may be important is that I think there is a fairly considerable elevation in unesterified fatty acids with a meal. My question is this: does this influence albumin binding? Is this likely to be important?

Aldini: I think that the fatty acid may greatly influence the extent of the albumin binding with bile acids. We used a free fatty acid albumin preparation that resolves the problem. About the effect of the concentration of fatty acid on the albumin binding, I think that, in some physiological phases (i.e. during digestion) when the hepatic synthesis is activated and a lot of fatty acid in the blood is present, they may play an important role. Therefore, I think that some bile acids, more particularly cholic acid which is less tightly bound to albumin, may be displaced from albumin. In this case I believe that a faster uptake of cholic acid may occur. I do not think the same, for instance, for lithocholic acid. But if we consider that fatty acids are 99% bound to albumin and cholic acid is 45–50% bound, this may be a determinant of a more rapid cholic acid uptake during digestion.

La Russo: Albumin has a molecular weight of about 60 000, which means that if it is going to be taken up by the hepatocyte it would probably be taken up by the mechanism of endocytosis, perhaps by receptors. Do you know, Dr Aldini, whether or not the bile acid albumin in complex is taken up together by hepatocyte, or whether or not the binding takes place outside the hepatocyte and then the bile acid is released from the albumin? Do you have any data on the mechanism of uptake? Or if no data, do you have any speculation on what happens at the sinusoidal pole of the hepatocyte with regards to the protein bile acid complex?

Aldini: Such a problem is a very difficult one and I followed some papers which appeared recently in literature by Dr Forker (1981). I did some experiments increasing the albumin concentration in the perfusion media and I showed that there was a competitive inhibition of albumin on taurocholate uptake, in the sense that the maximal uptake velocity was not affected, but the K_m was increased about three times. Therefore, this may be interpreted as the fact that the same carrier is for albumin complex and for albumin alone. A possible speculation is that the particular carrier links albumin when the bile acid is taken up by itself. I know the paper of Anwer (1979). He told that he found that albumin presented a competitive inhibition of the taurocholate uptake, but not of the cholate uptake. Therefore he says that probably there are two carriers for the bile acids.

I think that, to date, the problem is very far from solution. But my personal feeling is that, while for some bile acids a receptor for albumin is very important for the uptake (I mean for lithocholic acid, which is almost completely bound to albumin), it may not be the same for taurocholic acid or glycocholic acid. Therefore, of the two components of the bile acid uptake, as well as of the fatty acid uptake, the exact role has to be quantitatively defined.

Paumgartner: We move on now to two very short presentations which both relate to the hepatic uptake mechanism. They relate to maturation of this mechanism during development and changes of this mechanism in old age. Dr Balistrieri will provide data on maturation of hepatic bile acid uptake mechanisms; then Dr Angelico will talk about old age; and Dr Molino will summarize these findings, and this will conclude the first part of the workshop.

Balistrieri: In terms of the determinants of the serum bile acid levels we can gather some very important clues as to the rate-limiting steps through study of the immature liver. As you know there is a period of 'physiologic cholestasis', or more appropriately, physiologic 'hypercholanaemia'. This was initially shown by the Bologna group and has been verified in several centres.

I would like to show you some of the data we have gathered and then make one or two comments regarding our speculations. Figure 8 shows the data that we obtained through study of mothers and their infants in the first few days of life. What we have shown here is the concentration of bile acids, in micromoles per litre, the mean plus or minus the standard error of cholylglycine measured by RIA and conjugates of chenodeoxycholate measured again by RIA. As you can see, compared to maternal levels (50 mothers), the cord levels were very low, but within the first day of life there was a rise noted in the 69 infants in which cholylglycine was measured. This rise continued throughout the first 4 days of life. This might bring to mind the analogy of physiologic hyperbilirubinaemia, however, the elevated levels persisted throughout the first 4–5 months of life.

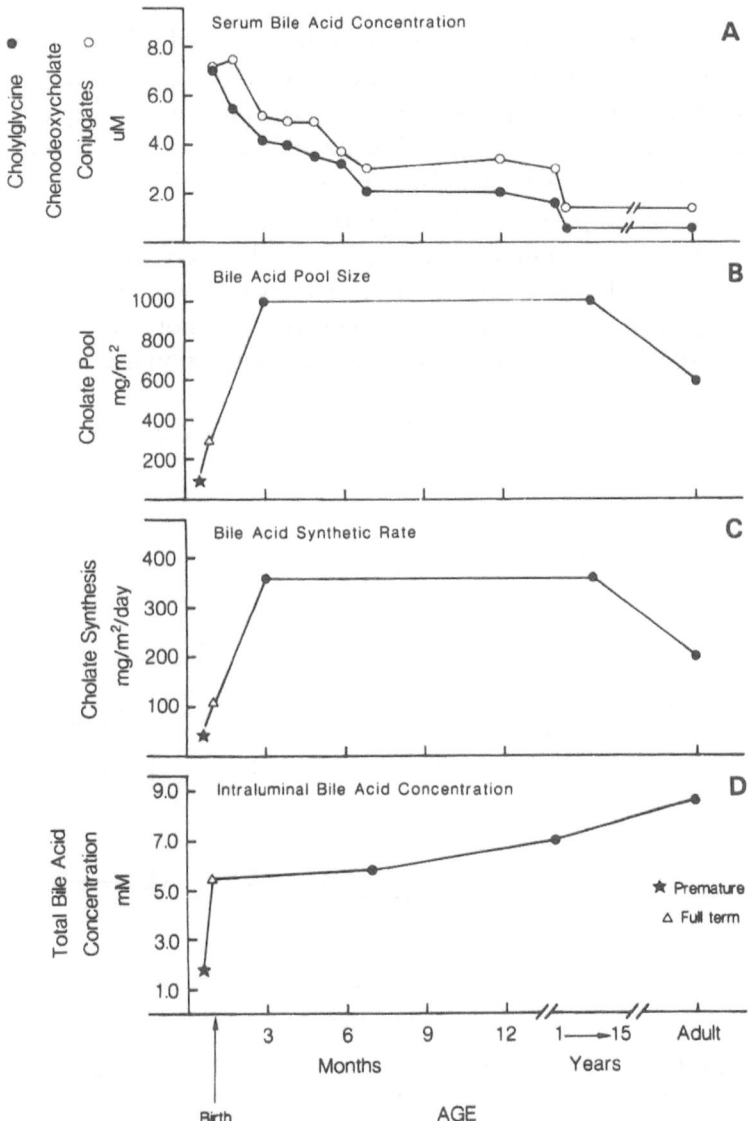

Figure 8 Graphic depiction of compiled data regarding the development of changes in various aspects of bile acid metabolism in humans. **A:** Progressive decline on the serum concentration of the primary bile acids (cholylglycine and conjugated chenodeoxycholate) with age (Suchy *et al.*, 1981). **B, C:** Bile acid kinetics studied by isotopic dilution reflected in bile acid pool size and bile acid synthetic rate; data from premature and full-term neonates from Watkins *et al.* (1973); data from infants and older children from Heubi *et al.* (1982); data from adults from Vlahcevic *et al.* (1971). **D:** Total bile acid concentration in duodenal samples; data in premature and full term neonates from Watkins *et al.* (1973); data from infants and older children from Heubi *et al.* (1982); and data from adults from Porter *et al.* (1971)

35

We now have shown, through measurement of both the fasting and postprandial levels of cholylglycine and conjugates of chenic, that the infant has a period of physiologic hypercholanaemia throughout early life. This physiologic hypercholanaemia is also manifested as an exaggerated postprandial rise (Fig. 9). If we look at the response to a meal over a period of three hours in normal children, as you can see, there is, of course, a rise in serum cholylglycine levels. In the infants, the level is not only higher to begin with, but there is an exaggerated postprandial rise. Tomorrow, we hope to discuss some of the specific phases of the enterohepatic circulation in the rat to show that uptake is indeed impaired.

I think that two points need to be made in follow-up of Dr Aldini's presentation.

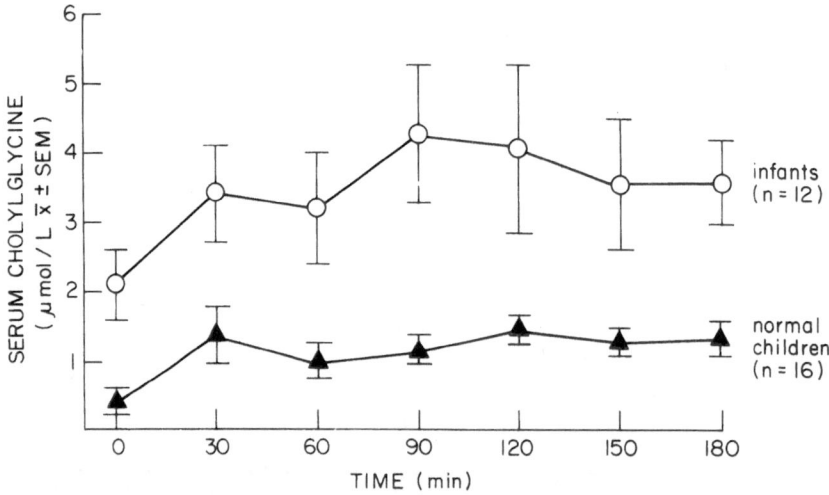

Figure 9   Change in serum concentrations of cholylglycine in response to a meal stimulus in normal infants and children

(1)   There may be, in early life, a difference in bile acid binding to albumin. This has certainly been shown for bilirubin and by the Bologna group in Gilbert's syndrome in which there is a moderate degree of bilirubin elevation. This may draw an analogy to the infant in which physiologic hyperbilirubinaemia may be present.

(2)   The blood flow or other perfusion factors may be quantitatively different in early life.

36

I hope to show you more about the immaturity of the enterohepatic circulation, and pinpoint specific rate-limiting phases.

Paumgartner: Now Dr Angelico, can you tell us something about what happens in old age?

Angelico: My contribution does not relate to old age, but to the effect of ageing on serum bile acids.

Within the previously mentioned epidemiological study on the prevalence of gallbladder diseases in a femal population (GREPCO), we have correlated the fasting serum primary bile acid levels with age. Figure 10 shows the mean levels of serum bile acids according to age decades. The mean bile acid values were within the normal range in all the age groups. Only 18 females in this study showed pathological results, and were homogeneously distributed according to age. As you can see, we found higher serum bile acid levels with increasing age. The difference between 20- and 29-year-old females and females in other age groups is statistically significant.

A positive linear correlation between serum bile acids and age was present. However, when we performed a multiple linear regression analysis including other parameters, such as age, body mass index, SGPT, and serum lipids as independent variables, and serum bile acids as dependent variables, this correlation (Fig. 10) was present no more. A highly positive correlation was found between serum bile acids and SGPT, which, interestingly, was also present excluding those females with abnormal results. Surprisingly, we found a negative correlation between serum bile acids and total serum cholesterol and a positive correlation with high-density lipoprotein cholesterol and serum phospholipids.

While the correlation with SGPT might be obvious, the correlations with serum lipids are very unclear and I present them to the audience as a matter of speculation. One possible explanation could be that at least a part of serum bile acids are transported in health by HDL-lipoproteins.

Paumgartner: These are very interesting data, and remind me of the data from the Mayo Clinic which show that patients with hypercholesterolaemia of type 2A have lower bile acid levels in serum than healthy subjects. Have you had some patients with hyperlipidaemia in your groups?

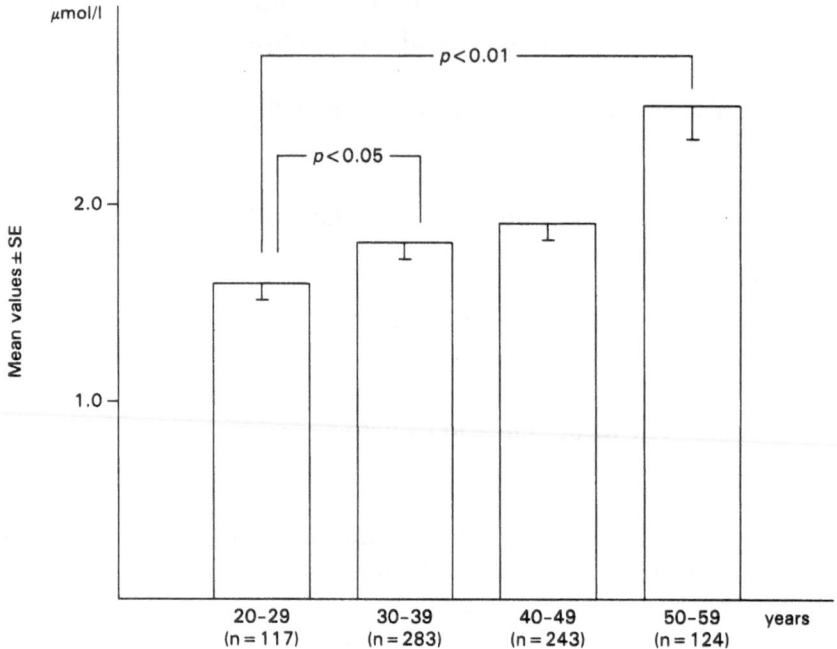

Figure 10 Fasting serum bile acid levels according to age classes in 767 females (cholecystectomized subjects excluded)

Angelico: The prevalence of hyperlipidaemia in this study was very low and the correlations between serum bile acids and serum lipids are still present also excluding hyperlipidaemic females from the statistical analysis.

Table 3 Multiple linear regression analysis between total fasting serum bile acid levels and other seven variables, in 807 females (cholecystectomized subjects excluded)

	T-value	p
Age	1.60101	n.s.
Body mass index	1.22181	n.s.
SGPT	4.97246	<0.001
Total serum cholesterol	− 2.16881	<0.05
HDL-cholesterol	2.186	<0.05
Serum triglycerides	1.80007	n.s.
Serum phospholipids	2.28622	<0.05

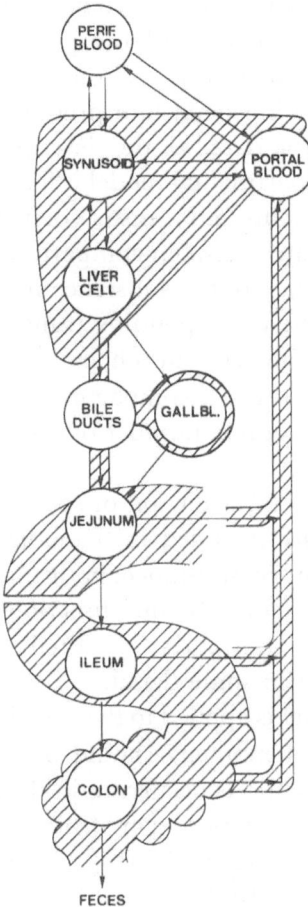

Figure 11 Depiction of anatomical spaces and functional connections of the model describing the enterohepatic circulation

Paumgartner: We shall now go on to the last presentation, in which Dr Molino will bring all these difficult problems together into one model and will give us an overview on what happens with bile acids in the enterohepatic circulation and how they influence serum bile acid levels.

Molino: The model I will now present describes the metabolism and enterohepatic circulation of bile acids. It is the result of a collaboration between mathematicians and physicians of the Torino group and Dr Alan Hofmann.

Two main aspects were considered in developing the model. First, a detailed definition of spaces and transports, on the basis of anatomical and functional considerations; second, the choice of suitable mathematical methods giving good interpretative and predictive results without sacrificing the detail of the description.

In general, a compartmental model is formed by block and arrows indicating compartments and transfer coefficients, respectively. Any movement of substance between compartments can be computed as the product of the mass of the substance in the donor compartment times the value of the corresponding transport coefficient.

Bile acid metabolism and enterohepatic circulation are quite complicated processes, so that a compartmental model fully describing them should include a great number of compartments and transport coefficients.

Figure 11 is a general depiction of spaces and coefficients, which should be necessarily included in a model describing the enterohepatic circulation of any substance: both anatomical spaces (hepatic, biliary, circulatory, enteral) and functional aspects (circulatory, biliary and intestinal transports, intestinal absorption, liver uptake) are represented in it in some detail.

When such a model is applied to the description of bile acid metabolism, some other phenomena should be also taken into account, namely biotransformations occurring in the liver (conjugation) and in the intestine (deconjugation, dehydroxylation). As an example, for cholic acid, the following model (Fig. 12) should be used, derived from the previous one. In it, liver and intestinal biotransformations were suitably taken into consideration: as a consequence each anatomical space now consists of three compartments defined on a chemical basis and representing the unconjugated cholic acid and its tauro- and glyco-conjugated derivatives.

Let us now separately consider the main features of the model.

As concerns the liver compartment, both hepatic uptake and hepatic secretion into bile are described, and conjugation processes are also represented.

In the biliary district, the model separately represents a bile duct space and a gallbladder space. Variation of the gallbladder volume and output during the day are a well known physiological event: to represent these important facts the coefficients indicating transports between the two biliary compartments must then be made time-dependent.

40

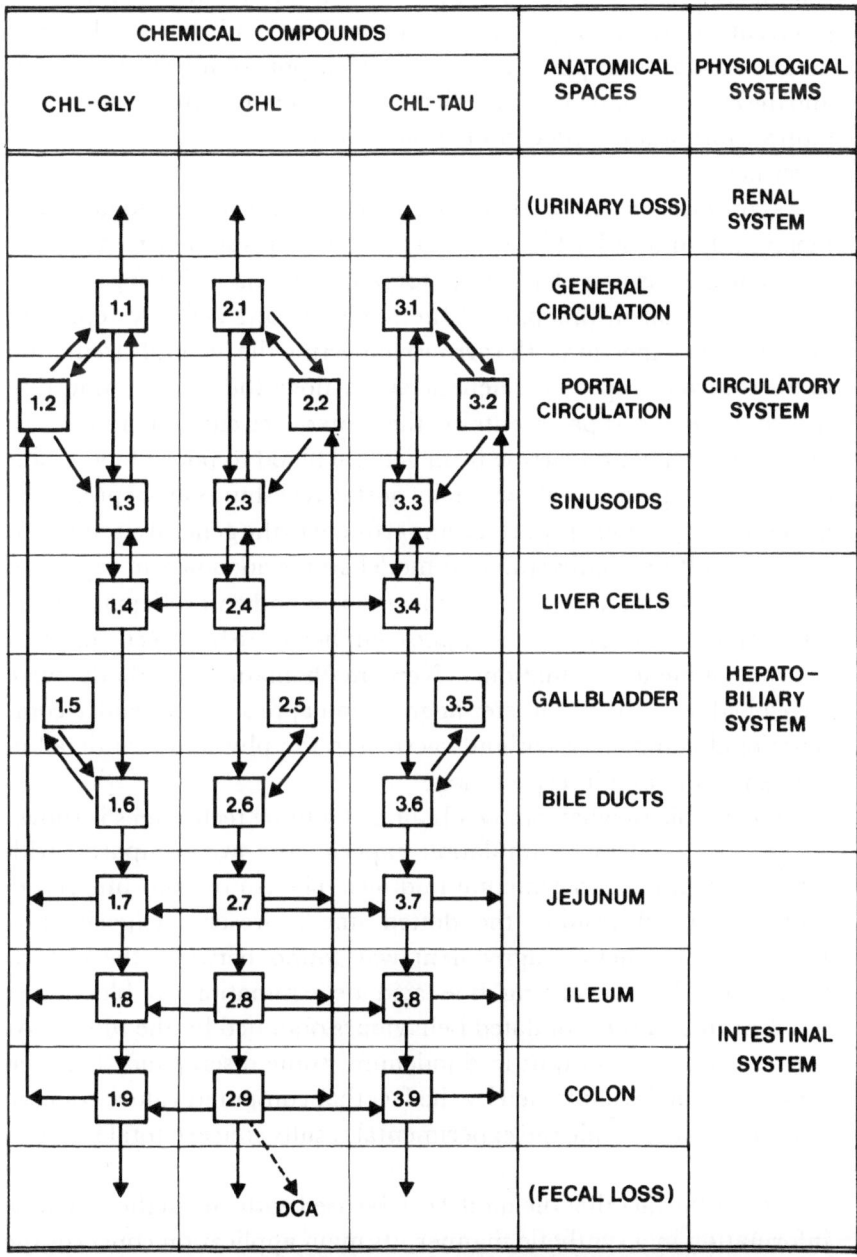

Figure 12 Compartments and transfer coefficients of the cholic acid model

Intestinal space is divided into three compartments (jejunal, ileal, colonic) to separately describe the events occurring in each intestinal tract. All intestinal compartments are connected with the portal tract to describe absorption phenomena. The transport of intestinal content and the faecal output are also indicated in the model. Finally, intestinal biotransformations (deconjugations, dehydroxylations) are also described.

As concerns the circulatory part of the model, general blood, portal blood and sinusoidal blood are separately represented to allow an adequate description of all circulatory phenomena. It is very interesting to note that in this part of the model arrows actually represent anatomical connections: the arrow connecting the general circulation to the sinusoids represents hepatic artery flow; the arrow connecting the sinusoidal compartments to the general circulation represents hepatic vein flow; the arrow from general blood to portal blood indicates mesenteric artery flow; finally portacaval shunts are represented by the arrow joining the portal compartment to the general circulation.

The resulting compartmental model seems adequate to represent the more relevant aspects of the metabolism and enterohepatic circulation of bile acids. However it is too complicated to be directly used for pharmacokinetic evaluations. New mathematical methods were developed (e.g. the parameter aggregation approach) to reduce computational complexity without sacrificing the physiological detail of both structure and interpretation.

An example of what can be obtained by these techniques is shown in Fig. 13, in which simulation experiments are compared with directly obtained experimental findings. The continuous line represents simulated results; the dotted line represents experimental results. A satisfactory agreement was found between the experimental results concerning bile acid determination in blood and duodenum and the simulated behaviours obtained by the model. As concerns bile acid output in duodenum, some discrepancy between the curves can be explained by the fact that computed values concern only cholic acid, while the experimental results concern total bile acid output.

Besides the fact that the model can be used with any of the available information in a synthetic manner, its main application concerns the possibility of using simulations to predict concentrations and behaviours in not easily accessible compartments. This might substantially improve pathophysiological information for both health

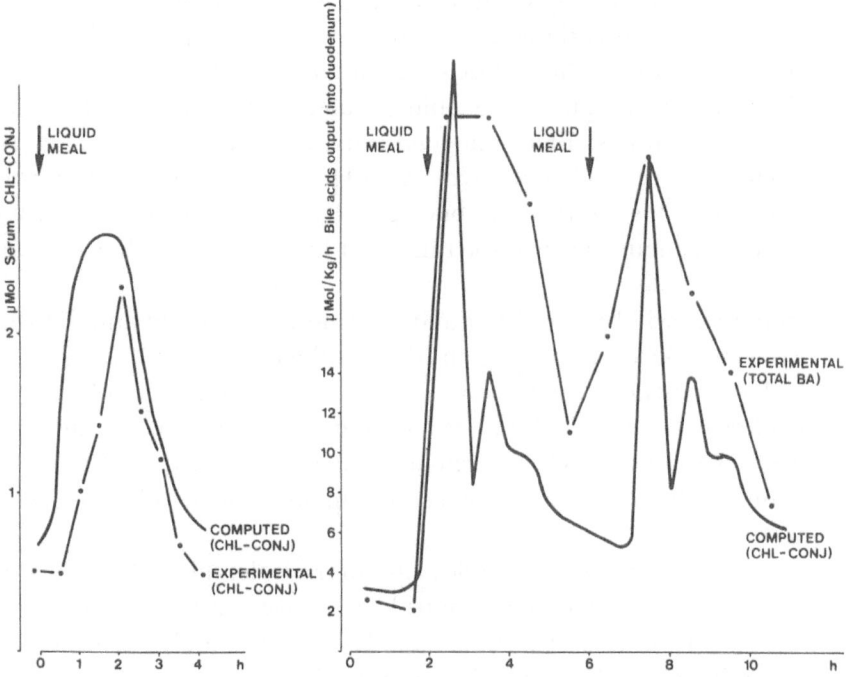

Figure 13   Comparison of the results obtained by simulation and original experimental data. *Left:* Serum levels of cholyl-conjugates (experimental data from La Russo *et al.*, 1978). *Right:* Hepatic secretion of cholyl-conjugates (experimental data from Van Berge Henegouwen *et al.*, 1978)

and disease conditions; moreover simulation studies might be very useful to aid in designing new experimental conditions.

Paumgartner: Dr Molino has shown that in the future we may be able to predict, if we know all the variables, what the bile acid level has to be in a given subject. This would be a large step forward.

PART II

Barbara: The second part of the workshop deals with the evaluation of the usefulness of serum bile acids. Since many methods of applying the test have been proposed, I think we had better begin by defining the most suitable of these.

We can divide the test into two categories: the first is the fasting test, the second is the load test (intravenous, postprandial or oral). In my opinion the fasting determination is probably now the test of choice for its simplicity, reliability, safety, and low cost. Therefore I prefer to discuss firstly the load tests, in order to identify the test of choice; I would like to invite Alan Hofmann to give a short introduction on his views about bile acid clearances and the rationale of the endogenous bile acid tolerance test in patients with liver disease.

Hofmann: I will be very brief and in some ways merely amplify what Professor Barbara has said in his introduction.

The question is, when do we measure serum bile acid levels? As Professor Barbara has said, the fasting state is most convenient and it is desired by the clinical chemist. As we discussed in Part I, with Professor Paumgartner, it reflects the spillover of an unknown fasting state load.

We can measure serum bile acids after meals; this reflects the spillover of an unknown endogenous load, or we can measure bile acids after an oral or an intravenous load. If we give an oral load this reflects the spillover of a known endogenous load, so at first glance this would seem to be the best measurement in principle.

The reason we can say that we need a load is that the serum level reflects the first-pass clearance, and this – so far – appears to be rather independent of load in health and mild liver disease. So the serum level is then directly proportional to the hepatic load, and to interpret the serum levels the load must be known and the load is unknown in the fasting state. We therefore have to decide on the fasting state.

If we say that an endogenous load is to be considered, this can be done with a test meal, but the load is not defined. It certainly requires intestinal transit and normal ileal function for the bile acids – trihydroxy acids – which are reabsorbed actively. So we could conclude from this argument that an exogenous load was superior.

There are really two kinds of exogenous loads. We began some years ago with the intravenous load. This is predominantly, initially, an arterial presentation into the liver. It will not detect shunting. It is not dangerous systemically, but locally one can have a problem injecting mass into the vein. The colyl-glycine which we used is not very sensitive. Dr Sama will present some work suggesting that unconjugated loads may be more sensitive. This may be because the

uptake by the liver has different mechanisms and uptake of unconjugated bile acids may reflect, in part, the absorptive surface for the
passive component. So the sensitivity may depend slightly on the kind
of bile acid.

Now we can give an oral load. This is influenced by gastric emptying and dissolution kinetics. It measures the first-pass clearance and
the approach, to date, has been to use a bile acid which is absorbed
passively in the duodenum and jejunum. The obvious candidates
initially have been chenodeoxycholic, ursodeoxycholic or possibly
deoxycholic acids. Of these, the simplest one to use is ursodeoxycholic
acid because there is less of this among the endogenous bile acids, and
since, as we have seen from Dr Setchell and others, there are always
levels of unconjugated endogenous chenodeoxycholic and deoxycholic acids; ursodeoxycholic acid would probably have the lowest
endogenous level, making it the best candidate for an exogenous load.

Testa: We have studied the differences between fasting (SBAf) and 2 h
postprandial (meal test, SBAm) serum bile acids (SBA), determined
enzymatically. Seventy-two patients suffering from chronic liver
disease were studied: 17 chronic persistent hepatitis (CPH), 32
chronic active hepatitis (CAH), 11 chronic active hepatitis with
cirrhosis (CAHc) and 12 cirrhoses (C) (Table 4).

Table 4 Fasting (SBAf) and postprandial (SBAm) serum bile acids in healthy
subjects and subjects with liver disease

Group	No. of subjects	SBAf (M ± SE)	SBAm (M ± SE)
Healthy	20	2.6 ± 0.6	2.9 ± 0.7
CPH	17	6.9 ± 1.9*	14.1 ± 3***
CAH	32	13.1 ± 2.6**	28.2 ± 5***
CAHc	11	34.9 ± 17.4*	62.6 ± 18.7***
C	12	63.3 ± 17.2***	87.7 ± 27.5***

*$p < 0.05$; **$p < 0.01$; ***$p < 0.001$

Both fasting and postprandial SBA levels increase progressively
with liver damage. Yet the frequency of change above the abnormal
limits increases significantly from CPH to cirrhosis (Table 5). Concerning sensitivity the meal test differs from fasting only in CAH
($p < 0.05$): probably this depends on saturation of the hepatic clearance by the endogenous load (Table 6). SBAm provides better

discrimination between CPH and CAH. SBAf is the most discriminant test for CAH, CAHc and C. To account for the observed differences between fasting and postprandial SBA, a regression analysis was performed between SBA, histology (score of necrosis, flogosis and fibrosis) and degree of portal hypertension (laparoscopic score) (Table 7). As the postprandial SBA have a significant relationship with histological pattern ($r = 0.35$; $p < 0.05$), the fasting SBA are not correlated ($r = 0.21$; $p > 0.05$). As the saturation of hepatic clearance by endogenous load seems to correlate meal test with histological damage, portal hypertension seems to be the major determinant of the fasting SBA.

Table 5 Sensitivity (%) of abnormal results of SBAf and SBAm in chronic liver disease

Group	SBAf	SBAm	p
CPH	17.6	47	n.s.
CAH	34.3	75	<0.005
CAHc	63.6	90.9	n.s.
C	83.3	100	n.s.
	$p<0.01$	$p<0.01$	

Table 6 Discriminant levels of SBA between various liver diseases

Group	Fasting DL (μmol/l)	TE%	Meal DL (μmol/l)	TE%
CPH/CAH	7.4	34.5	14.1	30.5
CAH/CAHc + C	20.6	33.5	40.8	35
CAHc/C	34.3	30.5	59.6	37

Table 7 Correlation index between SBA and histologic–laparoscopic findings

Score	SBAf	SBAm
Necrosis	0.22	0.36*
Inflammation	0.07	0.34*
Fibrosis	0.09	0.35*
NEC + INF + FIB	0.21	0.35*
Portal hypertension	0.36*	0.36*

*$p<0.05$

From these results it can be seen that, as far as enzymatic determination is concerned, postprandial SBA have greater sensitivity for detecting liver damage. The fasting SBA are more valid in discriminating liver diseases associated with portal hypertension.

We studied the diagnostic ability of the SBA versus some liver tests (ASAT, ALAT, GGPT, BSP test: retention to 45 min and uptake clearance) (Table 8). In discriminant analysis between chronic liver disease, the aminotransferases and SBAm provide better discrimination between CPH and CAH, SBAf remains the most discriminant test of CAH, CAHc and C.

Table 8 Discriminant analysis of SBA and 'liver tests' between various liver diseases

	CPH/CAH test		CAH/CAHc + C test		CAHc/C test	
	Lo	TE%	Lo	TE%	Lo	TE%
ASAT	14.3	28	42.7	49	41.5	46
ALAT	10.6	27	28.7	48	25.9	41
GGPT	60.2	36	106.1	47	108.5	44
BSPr	7.5	33	16.4	36	20.9	42
BSPk1	10.7	35	6.3	35	4.7	32
SBAf	7.4	34.5	20.6	33.5	34.3	30.5
SBAm	14.1	30.5	40.8	35	59.6	37

In a multivariate analysis (Table 9) the SBA, both fasting and postprandial, and the BSP test, both retention and clearance, have diagnostic value in discriminating between chronic liver diseases. There is evidence therefore that in screening of liver diseases, the SBA could substitute the BSP test.

Table 9 Discriminant analysis between various liver diseases with two groups of 'liver tests'

Groups	1			2		
	Lo	TE%	C%D	Lo	TE%	C%D
CPH/CAH	− 4.2	20.6	32	3.9	21.2	40
CAH/CAHc + C	− 1.2	31.1	93	− 5.1	32.3	95
CAHc/C	− 1.9	19.2	1	− 9.6	8.1	3

(1: ASAT, ALAT, GGPT, SBA; 2: ASAT, ALAT, GGPT, BSP)

Di Mario: The composition of the standard meal used in this study is shown below; this comprises egg and malt extract and sorbitol as sweetener:

Standard meal (50g)
Sorbitol
Dried yolk of egg
Malt extract

Figure 14 summarizes our results: in the vertical axis you can see the levels of total bile acids determined by Becton–Dickinson RIA expressed in micromoles per litre, and in the horizontal axis the groups of patients studied: 10 control subjects, 10 patients with chronic persistent hepatitis, 14 with primary biliary cirrhosis and 10 with liver cirrhosis. The serum levels of total bile acids before and 2 h

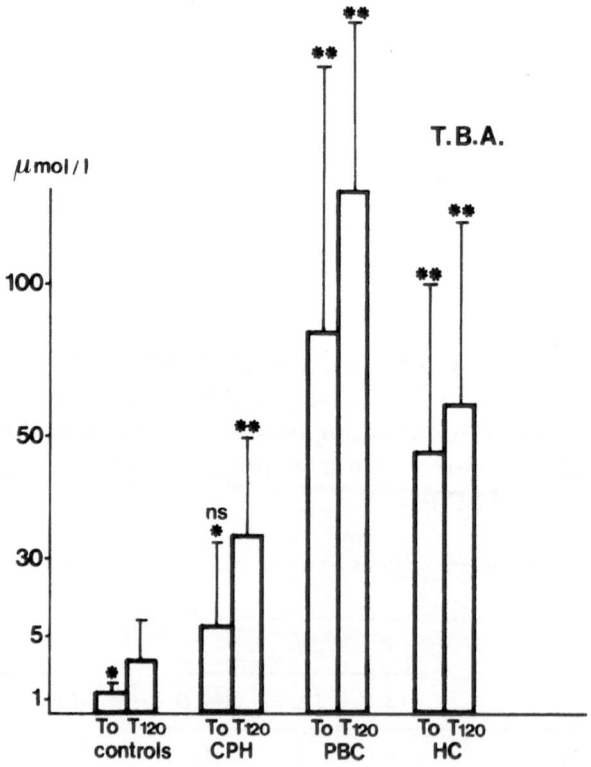

Figure 14 Total bile acid levels (T.B.A.), basal (To) and 120 minutes after meal (T120), in control subjects and in patients with chronic persistent hepatitis (CPH), primary biliary cirrhosis (PBC) and liver cirrhosis (HC)

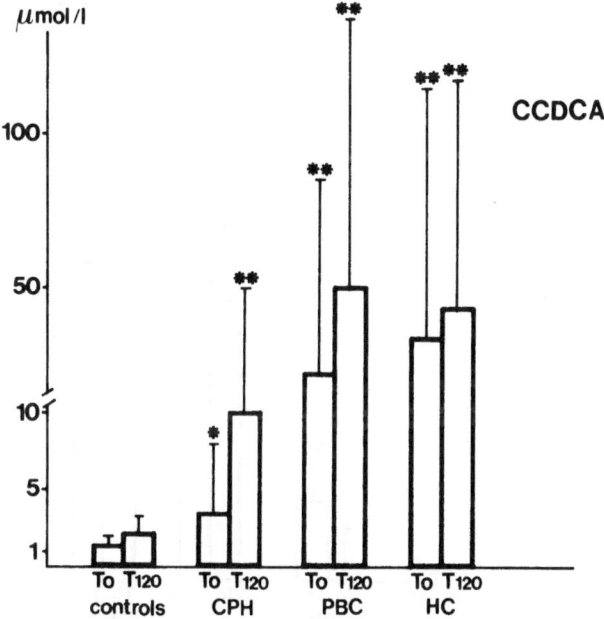

Figure 15 Conjugated chenodeoxycholic acid levels (CCDCA), basal (To) and 120 minutes after meal (T120), in control subjects and in patients with chronic persistent hepatitis (CPH), primary biliary cirrhosis (PBC) and hepatic cirrhosis (HC)

after the meal were evaluated. You can see a significant increase of serum bile acids 2 h after the meal in patients with chronic hepatic disease, particularly in patients affected by cirrhosis and primary biliary cirrhosis.

Figure 15 concerns chenodeoxycholic acid conjugates, determined by RIA: a significant increase was found 2 h after the meal for the patients with chronic liver diseases. Figure 16 shows the levels of the cholic acid conjugates in our material: you can see a significant increase both in basal levels and after a meal in patients affected by chronic liver disease.

Hofmann: I would like to make a comment about the whole problem of serum bile acid levels, because the problem is we are changing now from physiological science to another discipline which is the discipline of clinical chemistry or diagnostic chemistry. In science we are trying to compare groups and to find a difference between the groups which has some probability that the results are not due to chance, our p value. When we are working in testing, that is not enough, because

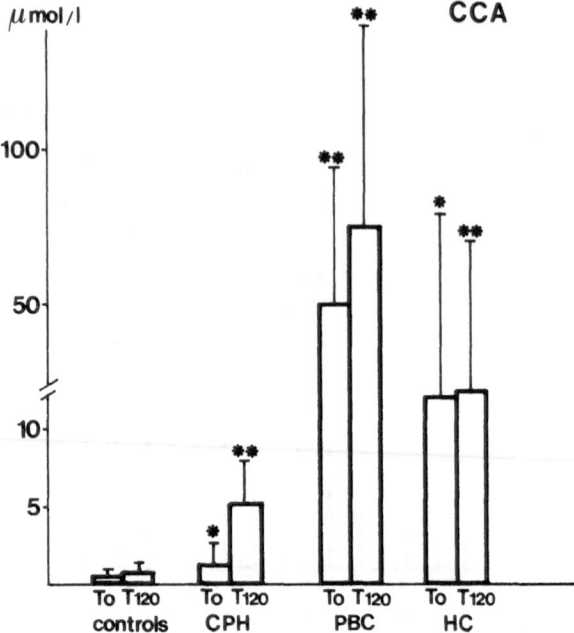

Figure 16 Conjugated cholic acid levels (CCA), basal (To) and 120 minutes after meal (T120), in control subjects and in patients with chronic persistent hepatitis (CPH), primary biliary cirrhosis (PBC) and hepatic cirrhosis (HC)

we can surely have differences between health and disease, but we demand much more of the measurement. We have to look at false-positives and false-negatives which become translated into the jargon of clinical chemistry, which is sensitivity and specificity.

So, unfortunately for most of us, who are not clinical chemists, we have to use a different way of thinking about our results, and we even have to express them differently.

The other comment that I would like to make is that the origin of the postprandial bile acid level reflected initially insensitive methodology. When Kaplowitz, Kok and Javitt (1974) on the basis of 10 patients proposed that the postprandial level was better, they did not know that there was an increase in the postprandial level in healthy people, because they could not determine it with their gas chromatographic method which, at that time, was not sensitive enough. If the first-pass clearance does not change with eating, then there is no theoretical reason why the postprandial levels should be more sensitive, but it means we have to consider other factors or our theory is wrong, or both.

Podda: I want to add a comment which I think might help to explain why in chronic liver disease with portal hypertension, Dr Testa did not find an increase in the postprandial state. In portal hypertension, gallbladder volume – according to studies we have now under way with the ultrasound determination of both gallbladder volume and contraction – the gallbladder volume tends to be lower and there is a high residual volume after meals. So the load may in fact be much lower than in patients without portal hypertension.

Dowling: I wonder if I could add a few comments to supplement Alan Hofmann's remarks. If we are talking about liver function tests we are talking about tests of an organ with multiple functions: a synthetic function, a transport function, a conjugation function and a detoxification function. Bile acid transport is simply the transport of one anion or substrate and, therefore, only one function. Perhaps in a meeting where bile acid experts are talking to bile acid experts, we ought not to become too narrow, and should try to keep a broad dimension, realizing it is naive to imagine that any one single parameter or any one aspect of hepatic function is going to act as discriminant for liver disease in general. I think there is a real danger from being too enthusiastic about measuring serum bile acids or bile acid transport. The clinical chemist wants to know whether or not serum bile acids are more sensitive than other indices of liver function which he can measure by running a serum sample through an auto-analyser – whether it is bilirubin, transaminase or alkaline phosphatase.

The results of many studies have shown us that serum bile acids perform well as a test of liver function, whether measured during fasting, or in 1 h or 2 h or postprandial samples as a 4 h postprandial integrated curve. The question is really whether, in an age where we are increasingly making tissue and anatomical diagnoses, there is still a place for convincing clinical chemists, and our clinical colleagues, that we really should be introducing serum bile acids (as opposed to some other test) in the diagnosis of liver disease. I think the case is marginal, but I would appreciate the views of others.

Barbara: Now Dr Molino will talk on 'Kinetics of postprandial serum bile acids'.

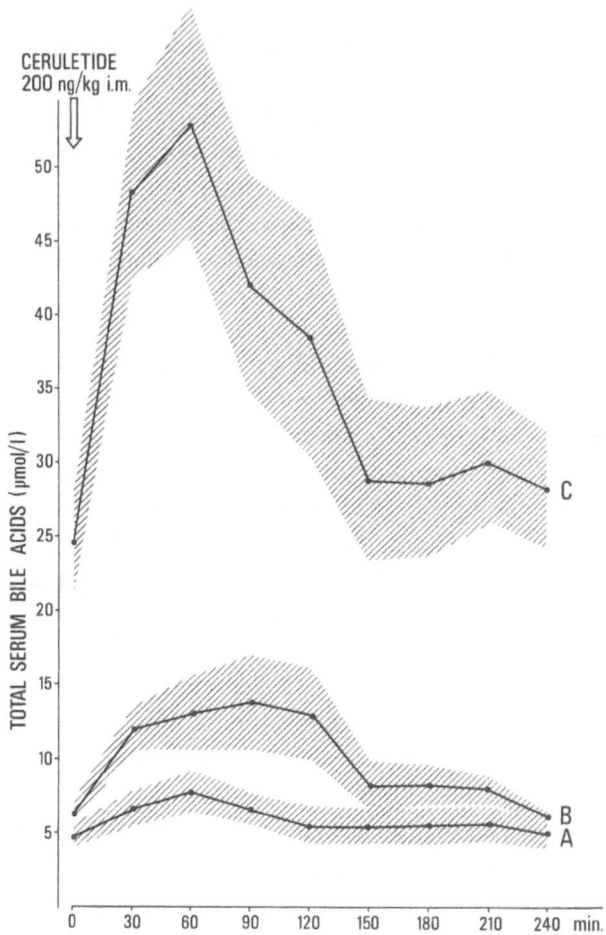

Figure 17 Blood kinetics of total SBA after C administration (MV ± SE). A = Normal subjects; B and C = chronic liver diseases

Molino: Blood kinetics of serum bile acids (SBA) after a standard meal or after the administration of an oral bile acid load was previously investigated by Matern and Gerok (1979). In those studies a late increase of SBA levels was sometimes observed, but never clearly explained.

In our department the blood kinetics of total and individual SBA was recently studied during a 4 h period after inducing gallbladder contraction by ceruletide (C) administration. This experimental model gave us the opportunity of investigating SBA kinetics under strictly controlled experimental conditions.

In the first 2 h period after C administration three types of behaviour were observed (Fig. 17). Normal subjects (group A) had
basal values of SBA not exceeding 10 μmol/l and peak values less than
12 μmol/l. The peak level was reached at about 60 min after C
administration, then SBA concentrations decreased, reaching basal
values at about 120 min. In liver diseases two different behaviours
were observed: some patients (group B) had basal values in the
normal range, but peak values exceeding 12 μmol/l; other patients
(group C) showed on the contrary abnormally high levels of total SBA
both in the basal condition and after gallbladder contraction.

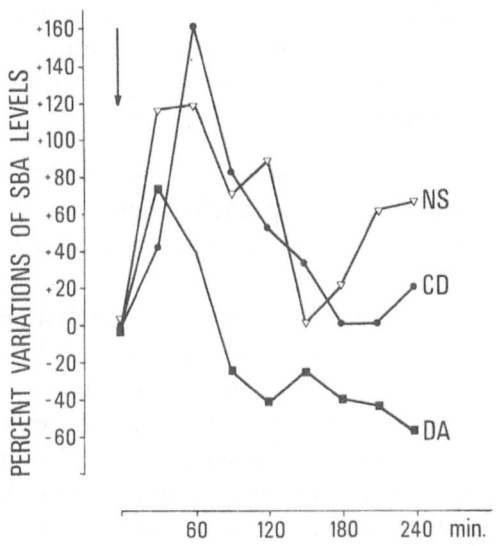

Figure 18 Typical examples of the different kinetic behaviours of total SBA in
pathological subjects, after C administration (see Text)

Moreover, when the whole 4 h period was considered, pathological
subjects showed three types of kinetic behaviour, which are exempli-
fied in Fig. 18. Type 1 (CD), in which, after reaching the peak level,
total SBA decreases to the basal concentration. Type 2 (DA), in which
the initial SBA rise is followed by the reduction to a concentration
lower than the corresponding basal levels. Type 3 (NS), in which the
curve is very similar to the first curve, except an evident late increase
of total SBA levels during the third hour, sometimes assuming a peak
shape, and also a momentary secondary increase at about 120 min.

53

The following additional experimental findings should also be outlined:

(1) the first peak was also found in cholecystectomized subjects, which suggests that the peak cannot simply depend on gall-bladder emptying;

(2) this first peak sometimes occurred quite early, within 15 min after C administration, too early to be attributed to the recirculation of bile acids released by the gallbladder;

(3) a momentary secondary increase of total SBA levels was sometimes observed during the second hour, at a time roughly corresponding to the expected enterohepatic cycling time-period;

(4) when individual SBA were measured, no significant increase of secondary bile acids was found corresponding to the secondary and late peaks, which is against the dependence of SBA kinetics on colonic absorption.

Our conclusions can be summarized as follows. The first peak occurring after C administration probably depends on the intestinal absorption of bile acids 'stored' in both the intestinal lumen and the gallbladder.

The persistence of high SBA levels after the first peak, besides an increased spillover due to the impaired liver uptake, might depend on the enterohepatic recycling of a greater bile acid intestinal load.

The following over-decrease of SBA concentrations might be related to an abnormal motility of either the gallbladder or the intestine.

The late peak observed in some patients cannot be easily interpreted: it might be referred to some events occurring in the biliary system and/or the intestine during liver diseases, such as the saturation of the storage capacity of the gallbladder or a secondary gallbladder contraction.

In any case our data show that, both in fasting conditions and after gallbladder contraction, SBA levels can be largely influenced by different extrahepatic factors, altering to some extent the actual bioavailability of recycling bile acids. These facts could significantly affect the diagnostic value of SBA determination in the evaluation of liver diseases.

I would also emphasize that these findings are a good example of what could be done by compartmental analysis of biological phenomena in order to validate pathophysiological interpretations of experimental data. In this case different simulations based on alternative pathophysiological hypotheses might be performed with the model for bile acids metabolism I presented before, and the comparison of the results obtained in different simulation conditions with the experimental findings could in fact be very useful in evaluating the adequacy of the underlying pathophysiological interpretations. Work is in progress in our department on these interesting problems.

Barbara: Professor Paumgartner will now talk about 'Postprandial comparisons between different methods'.

Paumgartner: As Dr Hofmann has said, from a theoretical point of view one would expect that fasting and postprandial serum bile acids (SBA) have equal sensitivity for detection of liver disease. The first-pass clearance of bile acids is reduced both in the fasting state and in the postprandial state.

If – as we have discussed – fractional hepatic uptake of bile acids does not change during meals, at least in normals and in patients with mild to moderate liver disease, it is surprising that several groups have in the past found a higher sensitivity of postprandial than fasting SBA for detection of patients with liver disease.

This finding could not be confirmed by others, including the Bologna group and the group at the Mayo Clinic. If one looks at the reports of the various groups it becomes apparent that the difference in methodology may have played an important role in these differences in clinical sensitivity.

In general, those who found an increased sensitivity of postprandial SBA have used an enzymatic or other rather insensitive methods for serum bile acid measurements. Thus, their conclusions may simply reflect difficulties of measuring small deviations from normal during fasting, a state in which bile acid levels are low.

To study this issue, Dr Mannes and Dr Stellaard from our unit have compared the sensitivity of fasting and postprandial SBA levels for detection of liver diseases in the same patients, using an enzymatic method and using a sensitive radioimmunoassay (RIA). The enzymatic method used was the assay of Nygaard, which gives comparable values to the enzymatic method we have developed ourselves in Bern. The RIA was from Becton-Dickinson, which mainly measures conjugated cholic acid and chenodeoxycholic acid.

We have performed this comparison in a group of patients with liver cirrhosis, documented by biopsy, who had normal transaminases. This group of patients often poses diagnostic difficulties and the liver disease is often missed if only the routine liver function tests are performed.

In a group of 29 cirrhotics with normal transaminases, there was a significant difference between the percentage of abnormal results between fasting and postprandial SBA levels, if the enzymatic assay was used. But there was no difference in sensitivity when the RIA was used. The RIA gave an abnormal result in 93% of cirrhotics with normal transaminases, both in the fasting and in the postprandial state. This shows that methodology is very important for the sensitivity of bile acid determinations for detection of liver disease.

If one now looks at the determinations by RIA and relates the fasting bile acid concentrations to the postprandial concentrations in the same patient, one sees what can be expected from theory, namely a fairly good correlation between fasting and postprandial SBA.

Festi: In order to evaluate whether or not postprandial SBA determination is more sensitive than the fasting one in detecting liver diseases, we studied 30 biopsy-proved liver disease patients (10 with chronic persistent hepatitis, 10 with chronic active hepatitis and 10 with cirrhosis) and 10 healthy subjects.

In each subject we measured, by specific RIA, serum levels of cholic (CCA) and chenodeoxycholic (CCDCA) acid conjugates in fasting state and after both a standard liquid meal and cerulein infusion ($2 \, ng \, (kg \, bw)^{-1} min^{-1} \times 5 \, min$) and serum levels of ursodeoxycholic acid (UDCA) after a 300 mg UDCA oral load. Table 10 shows the number of the subjects correctly allocated by a computerized procedure into each group on the basis of the different bile acid tests.

Table 10 Number of subjects correctly allocated by means of fasting and postprandial serum bile acids

	CCA		CCDCA		UDCA
	Meal	Cerulein	Meal	Cerulein	
F	19	22	18	24	16
2 h	21	25	20	24	18
MPPP	21	26	18	22	21
AUC	23	19	19	25	17

F   = Fasting
2 h   = 2 Hours after stimulus
MPPP = Maximal postprandial peak
AUC = Area under the curve

Our data suggest that the oral bile acid load, either obtained by a standard meal or cerulein infusion, or by UDCA administration, is not significantly more sensitive than the fasting bile acid determination. The few cases of correct allocation gained by the bile acids load, in our opinion, do not justify the use of this method rather than the more simple fasting determination.

Furthermore there are several problems with the standardization and interpretation of the bile acid load. The great variability of the mean time of the maximal postprandial peak (Table 11), and therefore the need of a prolonged blood sampling, is the main disadvantage of the bile acid load; while the UDCA tolerance test performed by the administration of gelatine tablets is influenced by gastric emptying.

Table 11 SBA Loads: mean time (and range) of the maximal peak

	CCA		CCDCA		UDCA (Oral load)
	Meal	Cerulein	Meal	Cerulein	
Normals	86 (10–180)	74 (4–180)	112 (15–180)	52 (10–180)	172 (165–180)
CPH	126 (60–180)	94 (60–135)	106 (30–180)	66 (15–135)	161 (45–180)
CAH	118 (30–150)	66 (15–180)	112 (75–165)	70 (15–180)	131 (30–165)
C	138 (75–180)	99 (10–165)	119 (30–180)	80 (6–135)	147 (135–180)

Attili: A short question for Dr Paumgartner. How did you define abnormality of fasting or postprandial, since this may influence your results of course? Was the increase the percentage increase of bile acids after a meal similar when using RIA or other enzymatic assays?

Paumgartner: The upper limit of normal was taken as two standard deviations above the mean for our fasting and postprandial levels. The levels increased about two-fold after meals in both normals and patients with liver disease. The percentage increase was not significantly different in the group of normals and in the group of patients, and it was not helpful in differentiating between these two groups. It was larger with the RIA than with the enzymatic assay.

Chadwick: Since the fasting serum bile acid level is presumably dependent on gallbladder function during fasting, and since, when you take a meal, the gallbladder contracts, is there a theoretical reason why postprandial bile acid levels might discriminate better in liver disease?

Paumgartner: I would not go along with your first statement that in the fasting state the bile acid level in serum depends on gallbladder contraction. It depends on the interdigestive delivery of bile into the duodenum, and it has been shown that this is related to the interdigestive motor complex. In the fasting state there is intermittent delivery of bile into the duodenum. However, this is not necessarily related to gallbladder contraction. It could represent bile secreted by the liver which bypasses the gallbladder.

Anyway, you have a certain load of bile acids in the fasting state and there is no reason to believe that the fractional removal of this load in the fasting state is different from the fractional removal when the gallbladder contracts and the liver receives a larger load. The findings so far substantiate the contention that in normals, and in patients with mild to moderate liver disease, the hepatic uptake mechanism is not saturated.

Chadwick: That is not the point of contention. The point of contention is simply that gallbladder emptying does occur in the fasting state. It's very variable between individuals and therefore in any patient group you would expect a variable factor to be introduced into your calculation there. I do not argue with the hepatic uptake.

Paumgartner: The delivery of bile into the duodenum during the interdigestive state is intermittent but these fluctuations were fairly constant in absolutely fasting patients. One can expect that the amount of bile reaching the duodenum during an interdigestive period in a given subject is fairly constant.

Barbara: We must now discuss bile acid clearances, and Dr Sama will talk about the discrimination capacity of bile acid clearance within liver diseases.

Sama: I am sure that many people think that bile acid clearances are out of fashion. Nevertheless I am going to present some unpublished data from our laboratory concerning the use of plasma disappearance of bile acids in the diagnosis of liver disease. Our results, in fact, are somehow different from those that have been published so far.

We have studied 100 control subjects, 50 patients with chronic active hepatitis and 30 patients with liver cirrhosis. We performed the plasma disappearance of three ^{14}C-labelled bile acids: cholic, glycocholic and chenodeoxycholic acids, according to the method of Cowen and co-workers, 1975.

We analysed the plasma disappearance curves using the transfer rates of a compartmental model. Data have been expressed both by means of the mathematical parameters of the biexponential curve and by means of the transfer rates of the compartmental model. To evaluate the diagnostic usefulness of the procedure, two different discriminant analyses have been applied: a Bayes allocation rule and a non-parametric method utilizing Kernel function.

We did not find any possibility of discriminating clearly between normal subjects and patients with liver disease when glycocholic acid was used. As far as cholic acid is concerned we found 17% of misallocation with the Bayes procedure and 39% with Kernel function (7% false-negative, 19% false-positive and 7% of misclassification between chronic active hepatitis and liver cirrhosis).

If we look at the data obtained using chenodeoxycholic acid we found 27% of misallocation with the Bayes procedure and 32% with the Kernel method (39% false-negative, 9% false-positive and 21% of misclassification between the two liver diseases).

So we conclude that, in our experience, the plasma disappearance of the two primary bile acids can have some clinical usefulness in the diagnosis of liver disease.

Dowling: I think these are interesting results and I think they have great strength from numbers and careful analysis. However, I have got to say that with much smaller numbers we did not find unconjugated ^{14}C-labelled cheno to have such good discrimination in liver disease. Peter Issacs and John Iser in our unit in 1976, I believe, were interested in why patients undergoing treatment with cheno have high serum bile acid levels. Was this liver disease induced by treatment? Or was it an artefact of feeding a bile acid? So we too looked at the plasma disappearance of ^{14}C-labelled cheno, and as a control we had 17 patients with biopsy-proven liver disease. In eight of those the plasma disappearance curves were completely normal; in other words, a 50% false-negative rate.

Sama: I wonder if you analysed the curve by compartmental model or using a mathematical method or just by looking at the K1 and things like that.

Dowling: No, I think there are difficulties in interpreting mono- and bi-exponential plasma disappearance curves, and to avoid that problem we used two parameters; that is, the percentage of the injected material remaining at 20 min and the $T\frac{1}{2}$. Both of those indices gave a comparable pattern of results with similar false-negatives.

Hofmann: Dr Sama, you did not give us the details of your analysis of the curve. I assume that you did not look at the species in the peripheral blood after you gave the unconjugated acid to see if you had reflux of conjugated bile acid out of the liver.

Sama: We did it, in fact, in some patients. We found that in patients with liver cirrhosis there was a good agreement when calculating reflux of bile acids from the hepatocyte to blood using the model or analysing the amount of conjugated labelled cholic acid in the peripheral blood after injecting unconjugated cholic acid.

Hofmann: My question is this: I mentioned that the reason why unconjugated bile acids are more sensitive may be because the mechanism of hepatic uptake is different. Obviously there is a second factor, namely the need to form the co-derivative and to amidate it with glycine or taurine. Could you sort out which of these two factors were important in giving you the diagnostic sensitivity?

Sama: In my opinion it was the uptake.

Barbara: Now Niels Tygstrup on some comments about serum clearances in pathology.

Tygstrup: I have been asked to comment upon use of bile acid elimination rate as liver function tests. To discuss this problem in some detail it is important to clarify what the test should be used for. In general we can distinguish between a diagnostic and a prognostic purpose. For the moment we can disregard the overlap between the diagnostic and prognostic approach caused by the prognostic implications of most diagnoses. We can simply consider the diagnostic process as an attempt to classify the disease of the patient, i.e. to decide whether he belongs to a given group of patient or not. The prognostic assessment, on the other hand, is based on an estimate of severity of the disease, normally in a patient in whom the diagnosis has already been made. Prognostic tests may be used to follow the course of the disease, deterioration or improvement, the needs for treatment and to evaluate its effect.

It appears from this that what we expect from the diagnostic test is a binary (yes/no) answer, while the prognostic test should be quantitative. The diagnostic test may be illustrated by a lamp and the prognostic test by a scale.

The classification process. Most tests, including those of diagnostic test from which a yes/no answer is asked, are reported quantitatively, i.e. they are continuous variables. They are converted to discontinuous variables by introducing a discrimination limit, meaning e.g. that higher values are called 'positive' and lower values 'negative'. The discrimination limit is chosen in such a way that it allocates a maximum number of subjects studied to the class to which they actually belong.

It is very rare that a test always allocates all subjects to the correct class. Some who have the diagnosis will have a negative test, i.e. be 'false-negatives', and some will be 'false positives'. The number of false-positives may be reduced by choosing a 'more abnormal' discrimination limit. This makes the test more specific, but simultaneously less sensitive because the number of false-negative classifications increases. It may also be made more sensitive at the expense of specificity.

A test will work well as a diagnostic test if the difference between the mean values of classes which should be distinguished is large in relation to the variation of the values within the class, i.e. if the values are clearly separated.

To evaluate bile acid as a diagnostic test we must answer three questions: (1) Which classes do we wish to separate by this test? (2) What are the mean values in these classes? and (3) What is the variation?

I cannot provide you with these answers, but from pathophysiological considerations and general experience I will expect that the postprandial rise in bile acids will be very sensitive to portosystemic shunts and that bile acid blood levels, or rather bile acid elimination rates, will be sensitive to cholestasis. Unfortunately each test will also be influenced by the other pathophysiological factor and therefore the actual diagnostic value only can be assessed under very accurately specified conditions. In this respect bile acid tests probably will work very much like the BSP retention test.

Quantizing liver function. To quantize liver function, e.g. for prognostic purposes, means to measure one or more of the functions performed by the liver and relate this measure to what we think it ought to be, or what it was earlier. Since the liver function mainly consists of metabolic processes, and since the production, uptake, and excretion of bile acids is considered an important metabolic function, measurement of this or these processes would appear to be a relevant quantitative measure of liver function.

Quantization of metabolic processes generally is made by determination of the rate of the process at standardized systems, a large number of factors influences the rate of a process, but in the body, as in the test tube, the concentration of the substrate is an important determinant.

The relation between substrate concentration and process velocity in most cases is described by the Michaelis–Menten relation shown

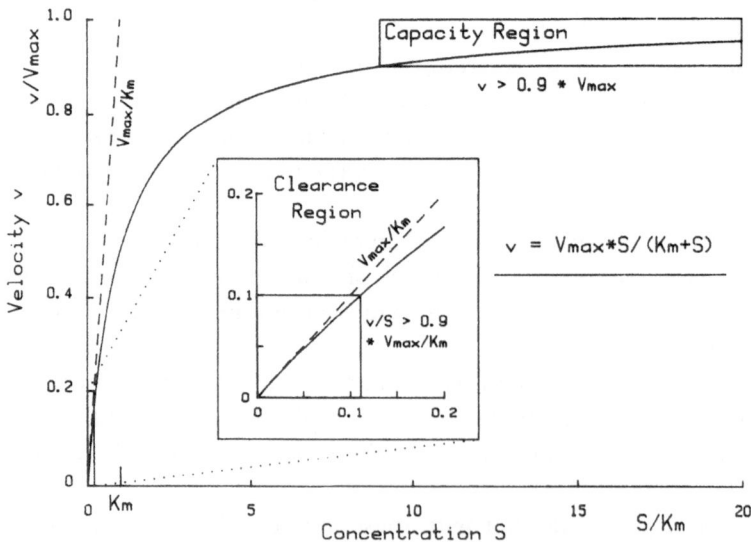

Figure 19 Regions of the Michaelis–Menten relation where functional assessment is simple, either because process rate (v) approximates Vmax (saturation region) or because clearance (v/S) approximates Vmax$/K_m$

in Fig. 19. Thus, if we can measure the rate of the process at a given concentration, and if we know what the rate should be at this concentration, then we can estimate if the function is reduced.

There is one problem, however. Since the curve is bent the substrate concentration must be reproduced with great precision to give comparable values of the rate of the process. Therefore it is necessary to use the extremes of the curve, i.e. the high *or* the low concentration range where the bend is less pronounced. These ranges, indicated in Fig. 19, are the capacity region and the clearance region.

The capacity region. In the high concentration range the velocity approximates the maximum of the process, the Vmax. This is in principle an advantage since this maximum may reflect the functional capacity of the liver or 'the functional liver mass'. It is only possible, however, if such high substrate concentrations are tolerated. It can be estimated that the saturation concentration of bile acid excretion is so high that it will cause serious side-effects, and that it therefore cannot be used under clinical conditions.

The clearance region. In the low concentration range the rate of the processes is approximately proportional to the concentration. The requirement is that the concentration is small in relation to the half-saturation concentration K_m. It can be derived directly from the Michaelis–Menten relation. Rearranging the equation for substrate concentrations approximating zero, i.e. much smaller than K_m, shows that rate over concentration, which is a clearance measure, equals the ratio between the kinetic constants Vmax and K_m.

Measurement of the clearance as the Vmax$/K_m$ ratio is also a useful functional estimate if it is assumed that only Vmax, the functional capacity, is changed by disease. K_m is a physicochemical parameter which may be assumed to be constant. Here we meet another complication, arising from the fact that we are working with a biological system and not with test tube observations.

If we look at the mathematically correct clearance expression (Fig. 20, eq. 1) which takes into account that the substrate *in vivo* is eliminated from blood streaming through the sinusoids of the liver, then we find that the rate of the process (v) depends on liver blood flow (F), in a rather complicated way. In other words, to measure clearance correctly we must also measure F, preferably by liver vein catheterization.

General clearance expression

$$v/S = F(1 - e^{-Vmax/K_m F})$$ (1)

Flow limited clearance

If $Vmax/K_m F \gg 1$, then

$$v/S = F$$ (2)

Enzyme limited clearance

If $Vmax/K_m F \ll 1$, then

$$v/S = Vmax/K_m$$ (3)

Figure 20 Clearance dependent on sinusoidal flow (eq. 1) and extreme ranges, where functional parameters may be estimated (eqs. 2 and 3)

Again we may look for the extreme ranges for simplification. This time it will be the extremes for the $Vmax/K_m$ ratio. It can be deduced from the correct clearance equation (Fig. 20, eq. 1) that if $Vmax/K_m$ is large, then the measured clearance will approximate F (Fig. 20, eq. 2). This clearance can therefore be used as an estimate of the hepatic blood flow which may be useful, but not so much for functional evaluation.

The other extreme where $Vmax/K_m$ is small leads mathematically to elimination of F from the equation and reappearance of the clearance equation given in Fig. 19 (Fig. 20, eq. 3).

Intuitively this is not surprising. The measured clearance of a substrate eliminated by the liver can never be greater than the hepatic blood flow irrespective of the true, enzymatic clearance ($Vmax/K_m$), and the smaller the latter is, the less will it depend on hepatic blood flow. This is illustrated in Fig. 21.

Bile acid clearance. Estimates of the $Vmax/K_m$ ratio of bile acid elimination indicates values of about 1 l/min in control subjects. It appears from Fig. 21 that clearance depends on flow in a rather complicated way in this region, as expected since a ratio is not very much different from the hepatic blood flow. Correct measurement of bile acid clearance therefore requires simultaneous determination of the hepatic blood flow, and this in most cases will mean that it cannot be accepted as a routine liver function test.

Conclusion. These considerations indicate that determination of bile acid elimination, by isotope methods or otherwise, is unlikely to be useful as a quantitative liver test for general clinical use. Also in this

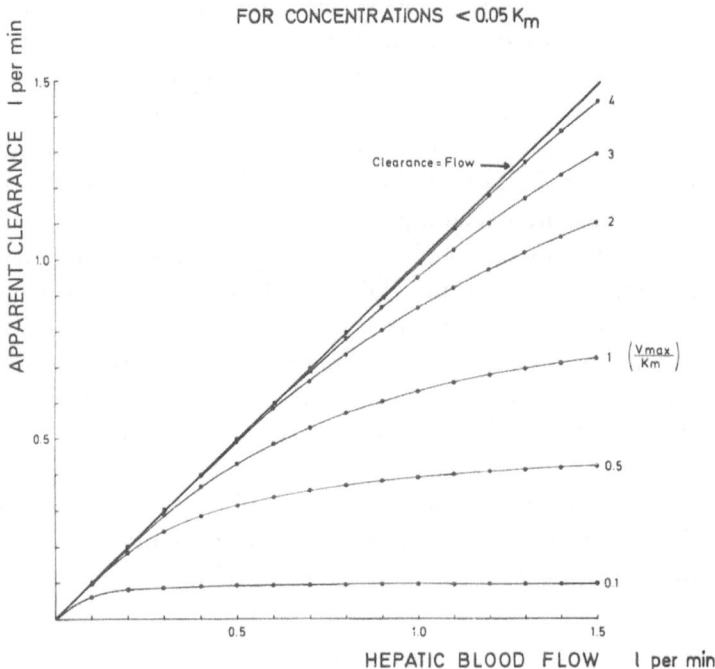

Figure 21 Relation between measured clearance and hepatic blood flow for substances with $V\text{max}/K_m$ ratio between 4 and 0.1

respect it is likely that a bile acid clearance determination will give practically the same information as the BSP clearance test, which has now been abandoned in most clinics. This does not exclude, however, the fact that other parameters of bile acid metabolism in the future may prove to serve this purpose.

Paumgartner: We have correlated postprandial bile acid measurements with various conventional liver function tests and with the BSP retention time. The only significant correlation that was found was with the BSP retention time. One would expect this on the basis of what you have just said. Both bile acid elimination and elimination of other organic anions depend on similar factors, on uptake function and excretory function. Therefore, it is not surprising that there is a correlation. This correlation, however, is not very close because of a number of other variables which influence the bile acid level.

Barbara: In summary the load test after *endogenous administration* of serum bile acid demonstrates a marked inter- and intra-subject variability. The AUC is probably the best way to express the results. It is important to standardize the type of stimulus. As far as the *exogenous loads* are concerned, the choice of UDCA is unsatisfactory (the solubility of UDCA in the intestinal lumen is low). However, this test needs sensitive techniques such as RIA or UDCA. The best way of administration is probably a bicarbonate solution and not capsules. A possible alternative to UDCA could be tauro-urso, which has a better solubility. Finally, the *clearances* have brought to light some problems with regard to their dependence on the liver blood flow and their potential dangerousness (particularly for tolerance and for radio-clearances). Their capacity to distinguish between various kinds of liver disease has not been well established. Therefore I would like to discuss the clinical usefulness of fasting serum bile acids in the detection, in the diagnosis, and in the management of liver disease. Is there anyone who has data on the specificity, sensitivity and predictive values?

Fiorentini: The aim of our work was to compare the diagnostic value of total fasting serum bile acids (tSBA), measured by enzymatic fluorometry, with that of fractionated serum bile acids, conjugated cholic (CCA) and chenodeoxycholic (CCDCA) acids, measured using a radioimmunoassay which was established in our laboratory in cooperation with Sorin Biomedica.

This work was performed on 88 normal subjects, on 118 patients without hepatobiliary diseases, but affected by other diseases and on 222 patients with hepatobiliary diseases. Cut-off values were considered 8.4 μmol/l for tSBA, 2.5 μmol/l for CCA and CCDCA. Using these cut-off levels tSBA had a 78% sensitivity, a 93% specificity and a 93% predictive value of a positive test, considering a 60% prevalence, which is the prevalence of hepatobiliary diseases in our gastrointestinal unit. CCA test had a 70% sensitivity, a 98% specificity and a 98% predictive value of a positive test. CCDCA had a 70% sensitivity, an 89% specificity and an 88% predictive value of a positive test; CCDCA specificity was significantly lower than tSBA and CCA specificity.

Our data show that radioimmunologically measured CCA has a positive predictive value which is higher than the other tests. On the other hand, tSBA measurement by enzymatic technique, which requires lower costs and times of performance, also has a 93% predictive value, that can be considered satisfactory in terms of cost–benefit ratio.

Barbara: How did you calculate the prevalence in order to obtain the predictive value?

Fiorentini: We considered the prevalence of hepatobiliary diseases in our gastrointestinal unit, where 60% of hospitalized patients suffer from hepatobiliary diseases. If we consider the 1% prevalence of hepatobiliary diseases, which is the value for the general population of our region (data for Piemonte obtained by Istat), we can calculate the positive predictive value of our tests, when used for screening for hepatobiliary diseases in the general population.

The correction of the positive predictive value for the 1% prevalence, using Baye's theorem, gives very low values of predictivity of these tests (10% for tSBA, 32% for CCA and 6% for CCDCA). Therefore the clinical usefulness of these tests resides in hospital practice: if a patient hospitalized in our unit has a tSBA value over the cut-off level he has a 93% probability of having a hepatobiliary disease; on the other hand, such a value in a person screened in the general population has only a 10% probability of reflecting a hepatobiliary disease. Predictivity of CCA is higher (32%), but a radio-immunological assay is not of practical employment in screening situations, due to its high costs of performance.

Festi: Serum levels of cholic, chenodeoxycholic and lithocholic acid conjugates were measured, by specific radioimmunoassay, in 322 biopsy- or peritoneoscopy-proved liver diseases and in 96 subjects without clinical and biochemical evidence of liver disease. In our population the sensitivity of SBA levels was 85% for cholic, 86% for chenodeoxycholic and 70% for lithocholic acid.

Orlandi: Let me emphasize here the distinction between the important pathophysiologic information we have obtained in past years through the study of bile acids in serum, in bile, or in urine and the problem of the rational use of serum bile acid determination (SBA) as a diagnostic test.

The diagnostic value of SBA depends basically on its simplicity, reproducibility, accuracy, sensitivity and specificity, and on a reasonable cost. Such requirements often show reciprocal influence. When we increase the sensitivity of a SBA method, for example, the specificity is likely to decrease. The sensitivity of a SBA loading test which requires multiple blood samples is higher than a fasting test, but the simplicity and the acceptability of the procedure becomes lower. The choice of a radioimmunotechnique can satisfy accuracy and sensitivity but involves the use of isotopes, a procedure which in medical care systems is usually reserved to departments of nuclear medicine, and implies the use of the test only when such facilities exist. The development of a simple and rapid bioluminescent technique, presented here by Dr Roda and co-workers, will allow a better compromise in balancing the above-mentioned requirements.

Such balance will depend on the specific purposes of each application of SBA tests, i.e. to screen for the presence of occult liver disease in the general population or in groups at risk of hepatic disease, or to attain or reject a diagnosis, or to provide prognostic information, or to assist in treatment.

The usefulness of SBA in screening for hepatic diseases, i.e. among people who consider themselves otherwise healthy, is uncertain. The Ancona Department of Gastroenterology has recently conducted a study of this type on an occupational population including 461 workers of the telephone company. The investigation has been based on postprandial SBA enzymatic fluorometric technique, which seemed a good candidate as screening method. We have observed a low specificity of the test as screening procedure and as 'case-finding' method in individuals with dyspepsia or minor digestive problems (Mosca *et al.*, unpublished data). Further investigations are needed in this field before assessing the real utility of SBA tests as a 'first-level' procedure. In this kind of observation the test can be influenced by unwanted bias, and can become somewhat different, as happens for most medical procedures when used 'in the field' for diagnosis or therapy of digestive diseases.

The clinical utility of SBA for diagnosis of liver diseases is better known. The SBA sensitivity in acute hepatitis, alcoholic liver injury, chronic hepatitis, and cirrhosis has been evaluated in some prospective studies and will be discussed. SBAD values are influenced by liver injury, alterations of hepatic uptake or transport of bile salts, of excretory function, of blood flow, and by portal-systemic shunting.

A different clinical utility of the test is therefore expected in distinct clinical situations. The 1978 Fogarty meeting on detection of hepatotoxicity due to drugs and chemicals included SBA among the tests potentially useful, but at that time its value remained to be established.

The criteria for accepting or rejecting a SBA test in terms of its clinical utility are very close to the criteria used for a trial on a new drug. First, the observation of a high sensitivity or other requirement in a series of patients with heterogeneous problems, including distinct type of liver injury, does not allow, per se, any conclusion about the clinical utility of the procedure. Such 'fishing expeditions' can only suggest that SBA could be a good candidate for further investigations in groups of patients showing a given, well-defined clinical situation and a reasonable homogeneity. Second, we have to demonstrate that in a given situation SBA is more useful than conventional tests, when used alone or in combination with other procedures, in a way similar to that needed to demonstrate that a new drug is superior to the old ones when administered alone or in combination with other drugs before marketing. Third, the goal of the test must be clinically relevant in preventive, diagnostic, prognostic, or therapeutic terms. The high sensitivity of a given test for detection of mild hepatic steatosis, for example, should be of little clinical value due to the irrelevance of a situation where therapy is not needed. On the contrary, the discrimination of a persistent form (CPH) from an active form (CAH) of chronic hepatitis satisfies most requirements for SBA utility assessment. At the moment such diagnosis implies invasive procedures such as needle liver biopsy, and the risk of side-effects of steroid treatments. Moreover, it is a frequent clinical situation.

Our experience in this field is briefly presented here in order to show some methodological problems. Table 12 shows the SBA values in a group of patients with CPH or CAH assessed by needle liver biopsy. In this series of patients SBA values were significantly lower in CPH than in CAH group ($p < 0.01$), but such a statistical evaluation was thought of little clinical relevance when deciding the right regimen in each patient. Only 5 out of 36 patients with CAH showed normal SBA levels, while 32 out of 67 patients with CPH showed SBA over the reference values (Table 12, part A). The sensitivity of SBA for the diagnosis of CAH appeared therefore reasonably high (86.1%), while its specificity was low (52.2%).

69

Table 12 Chronic hepatitis – serum bile acid level* total

	>1	≤1		
A.				
Active	31	5	36	Sensitivity 86.1
Persistent	32	35	67	Specificity 52.2
Total	63	40	103	
Predictive value	49.2 (PV +)	87.5 (PV –)		
CAH prevalence 35.0				

	>3	≤3		
B.				
Active	22	14	36	Sensitivity 61.1
Persistent	2	65	67	Specificity 97.0
Total	24	79	103	
Predictive value	91.7 (PV +)	82.3 (PV –)		
CAH prevalence 35.0				

*Times the upper limit of reference values (URV); PV + = positive predictive values;
PV – = negative predictive values

The best cut-off point was three times the SBA upper limit of reference values (URV). In this way (Table 12, part B) we could increase the specificity of the test to 97.0%, and the positive predictive value (PV + , i.e. the likelihood that the patient with SBA level more than three times URV actually had CAH) increased from 49.2 to 91.7% without affecting the negative predictive value (PV –) in a substantial way.

Incidentally, such values are less optimistic than our preliminary evaluations. This kind of discrepancy reminds us about the need of multiple investigations before attaining an adequate knowledge of a new diagnostic procedure, as well as showing that multiple therapeutic trials are needed for proper evaluation of new drugs.

It should be emphasized here that the evaluation of the SBA sensitivity and specificity, so familiar to us, are in fact a research task. These values are obtained in an investigation based on CPH and CAH which have been identified by an independent technique, i.e. liver biopsy. In medical care, on the contrary, we wish to use SBA tests without previous knowledge of histological findings, and SBA should serve to predict the likelihood that a given patient has (or does not have) CAH. In such investigations we have therefore to focus our attention on PV + and PV – values.

If we assume now that the results shown in Table 12 provide us with a proper evaluation of SBA test, could we suggest to general practitioners a high likelihood of CAH when SBA level is more than three times URV?

Table 13 shows how wrong such a suggestion could be. The PV + and PV – values shown in Table 12 were substantially dependent on the 35.0% prevalence of CAH among the examined patients, i.e. the prevalence occurring in a specialized department which acts as a tertiary care unit. In the primary care the percentage rate of mild forms of chronic hepatitis will likely be higher, and the prevalence of CAH lower, than in patients referred to a specialized unit. We can assume, for example, 1.0% prevalence of CAH (Table 13).

Table 13   Chronic hepatitis – serum bile acid level* total

	>1	⩽1		
A.				
Active	9	1	10	Sensitivity 86.1
Persistent	473	517	990	Specificity 52.2
Total	482	518	1000	
Predictive value	1.9 (PV +)	99.8 (PV –)		
CAH prevalence 1.0%				
	>3	⩽3		
B.				
Active	6	4	10	Sensitivity 61.1
Persistent	30	960	990	Specificity 97.0
Total	36	964	1000	
Predictive value	16.7 (PV +)	99.6 (PV –)		
CAH prevalence 1.0%				

*Times the upper limit of reference values (URV); PV + = positive predictive values; PV – = negative predictive values

In such situation the SBA sensitivity and specificity values will not change, while the PV + values will become respectively 1.9% (SBA >1 URV) and 16.7% (SBA >3 URV). This means that the general practitioner would use and interpret SBA values in a substantially different way than the specialist, due to the different patient population they have under care.

In conclusion, SBA tests should at present be used in specialized units and for the study of certain clinical situation such as cholestatic syndromes until *ad hoc* investigations show if and when they are useful in primary care, it is our duty, as hepatologists, to apply the clinico-epidemiological requirements as appropriate in order to avoid an otherwise predictable misuse of SBA tests in general practice.

Barbara: A brief comment: The comparison between healthy subjects and patients taken together, is not very useful from a clinical point of view. It would be better to consider each disease individually. Let us go on to discuss the discriminating capacity of serum bile acids, and the comparison between SBA and conventional liver function tests in order to assess the efficiency; in other words, to identify the reduced number of tests that produce no increased misclassification. In this part the first speaker is Fiorentini.

Fiorentini: In this study we compared the diagnostic value of total fasting serum bile acids (tSBA) with that of routine function tests (AST, ALT, G-GTP, bilirubin, alkaline phosphatase). These determinations were performed on three groups of subjects: group 1 included 97 normal subjects; group 2 included 187 patients without hepatobiliary disease, but affected by various medical disease; group 3 included 344 hepatobiliary patients, divided in various subgroups (moderate and severe parenchymal diseases, moderate and severe cholestatic diseases). Sensitivity, specificity and positive predictive values were calculated both for tSBA and for routine liver function tests. tSBA have a 78 % sensitivity, superior to that of the other tests, except for AST which has a similar value (74%). tSBA have a 93% specificity, with a value comparable to that of AST (92%).

Positive predictive value is 94% for tSBA and 93% for AST, considering a 60% prevalence of hepatobiliary diseases in our hospitalized patients. Reporting the predictivity to the 1% prevalence of hepatobiliary diseases, which is that of our region's general population, all tests have a very low positive predictive value (10% for tSBA, 9% for AST).

Since AST is a more practical test, with lower costs than tSBA assay, it can be considered the best diagnostic tool both in clinical and in epidemiological surveys.

AST can therefore represent the first approach to the subject with suspected hepatobiliary disease, while tSBA can be considered a second-level assay.

Combination of tSBA determination with another routine test of liver function can also be examined, in order to assess which combination gives the best improvement in diagnostic accuracy.

Testa: We studied the diagnostic ability of the SBA versus some liver tests (ASAT, ALAT, GGPT, BS test: retention to 45 min and uptake clearance) (Table 8). In discriminant analysis between chronic liver diseases the aminotransferase and SBAm provide better discrimination between CPH and CAH, SBAf remains the most discriminant test for CAH, CAHc and C. In a multivariate analysis (Table 9) the SBA, both fasting and postprandial, and the BSP test, both retention and clearance, have diagnostic value in discriminating between chronic liver diseases. There is evidence therefore that in screening of liver diseases, the SBA could substitute for the BSP test.

Di Mario: A very short report on the correlation between the levels of serum bile acids and serum bilirubin and aspartate-aminotransferase (AST) in chronic persistent hepatitis, primary biliary cirrhosis and liver cirrhosis (Table 14). As you can see there is a good correlation between serum bile acids and serum bilirubin in liver cirrhosis, and only for chenodeoxycholic acid, in primary biliary cirrhosis. For AST, a good correlation was also documented in liver cirrhosis and in chronic persistent hepatitis with bile acid levels.

Table 14 Correlation between total bile acids and other liver function tests

	TBA	*CCA*	*CCDCA*
Total bilirubin			
PBC	0.160	0.001	0.710***
HC	0.900***	0.80**	0.820***
CPH	− 0.06	− 0.19	− 0.270
AST			
PBC	0.292	0.179	0:160
HC	0.689*	0.795***	0.749***
CPH	0.956***	0.886***	0.975***
GGT			
PCB	0.096	− 0.12	− 0.099
HC	0.760**	0.64*	0.690*
CPH	0.290	0.190	0.340

$*p < 0.05$; $**p < 0.01$; $***p < 0.001$; no symbol: $p > 0.05$

Mazzanti: The aim of our research was to compare the behaviour of fasting and postprandial serum bile acids with other liver function tests, especially the percentage of BSP retention in patients with various types of chronic liver disease. The comparison between BSP and bile acids, especially postprandial, was carried out in order to see if there could be an alternative test to BSP in the monitoring of the treated and untreated chronic liver disease patient, considering the possible risk of allergies caused by the exogenous dye.

Serum total bile acids determinations were carried out in 161 cases, using the enzymatic–fluorometric method (Stereognost 3-alfa Flu). 136 patients suffered from various types of chronic hepatitis with and without cirrhosis (26 chronic persistent hepatitis, 54 chronic active hepatitis, 56 active cirrhosis) and 25 patients, without liver diseases and cardiocirculatory failure were used as controls.

The diagnosis was based on various laboratory tests and hepatic liver biopsy. Statistical analysis of the results was carried out by means of analysis of variance and Duncan's test (5%). The correlation coefficient between BSP and fasting and postprandial serum bile salts was also calculated. Our results show that there is a statistically significant correlation between fasting and postprandial serum bile acids behaviour and BSP retention in all our patients considered as a single group regardless of the different types of liver diseases (Table 15). These results confirm that serum bile acids assay is a sensitive test and that the behaviour of this parameter, especially postprandial, is similar to that of BSP retention. In conclusion, it seems possible to say that the bile acid postprandial test provides a valid alternative to BSP retention, which can carry dangerous side-effects, in monitoring chronic liver diseases.

Table 15

	Cases	BSP–FSBS	BSP–PPSBS
(A) CPH	26	$r = 0.36$ (n.s.)	$r = 0.433$ (n.s.)
(B) CAH	54	$r = 0.10$ (n.s.)	$r = 0.499$ ($p < 0.01$)
(C) Cirrhosis	56	$r = 0.42$ ($p < 0.01$)	$r = 0.493$ ($p < 0.01$)
(A) + (B) + (C)	136	$r = 0.49$ ($p < 0.01$)	$r = 0.510$ ($p < 0.01$)

CPH = Chronic persistent hepatitis
CAH = Chronic active hepatitis
BSP   = Bromosulphophthalein
FSBS = Fasting serum bile salts
PPSBS = Postprandial serum bile salts

Festi: We studied patients with biopsy-proved hepatic fibrosis (F), steatosis (S), chronic persistent hepatitis (CPH) (all considered as a single group of mild liver diseases: MLD), with chronic active hepatitis (CAH) and with liver cirrhosis (C). In all the considered liver diseases, fasting SBA resulted significantly different from normal subjects ($p < 0.001$). As far as the comparison between liver function tests (LFT) and SBA is concerned, we tried to identify the minimal number of tests necessary to reach the sensitivity of all the considered tests (Table 16). In MLD the overall sensitivity was 91.8% and four tests were sufficient to reach this value; in CAH, 100% of sensitivity, three tests; in C, 100% of sensitivity, two tests. In order to better define the discriminant capacity of SBA determination we performed a computerized analysis. Ing. Morselli will illustrate the results.

Table 16 Minimal number of tests necessary to obtain the maximal value of sensitivity

MLD: 91.8% – 4 tests	*C: 100% – 2 tests*
CCA + CLCA + SGOT + γ-GT	CCA + 1 L.F.T.
CCA + CLCA + SGPT + γ-GT	CCDCA + SGOT
CCDCA + CLCA + SGOT + γ-GT	CCDCA + SGPT
CCDCA + CLCA + SGPT + γ-GT	CCDCA + Bilirubin
CCDCA + CLCA + γ-GT + Bilirubin	CCDCA + Quick
	CCDCA + γ-Globulin
CAH:100% – 3 tests	CLCA + SGOT
CCDCA + γ-GT + Albumin	SGOT + Quick
CCDCA + γ-GT + γ-Globulin	
CLCA + SGOT + Albumin	

Morselli Labate: We have applied the discriminant analysis proposed by the Statistical Package for Social Science. Such a procedure allows one to assign the subjects under examination to one of the considered groups on the basis of the parameters studied. Cholic acid has presented the highest percentage of overall correct allocations (65.3%) in comparison to chenodeoxycholic (61.4%) and lithocholic (57.1%) acids. The normal subjects have been well identified (91.4%). This is a trivial result belonging to the criteria of normality that we have chosen.

Furthermore, the identification of liver diseases resulted to be quite satisfactory (chronic active hepatitis: 73.5%; cirrhosis: 64.4%), while the mild liver diseases have been almost completely misallocated (27.1% of correct allocations).

Considering more than one serum bile acid, there was only a slight increase of the percentage of correct allocations. With two bile acids, the best result has been obtained with cholic and lithocholic acids together (69.6%). A similar value has been obtained with all the three bile acids (70.1%).

The second step of our work has been to compare conventional liver function tests and serum bile acid levels. Considering the liver function tests alone, the 75.4% of correct allocations has been obtained, while a value of 79.6 has been reached when liver function tests and serum bile acid levels have been considered together. It should be noted that in the latter analysis, after cholic and lithocholic acids entered the stepwise procedure, the program has excluded chenodeoxycholic acid because it did not add any further information. In order to better define the role of serum bile acid levels, we have performed a factor analysis. Such a procedure enables us to see whether the information contained in the 11 biochemical analyses (serum bile acids plus liver function tests) can be related and summarized into a reduced number of dummy variables called 'factors'. Since the procedure does not need either the diagnosis or information about the nature of the biochemical tests, factors prove to be mathematical parameters and the results of the analysis depend only on the distribution of the data.

The procedure has identified two factors sufficient to explain the variance of the overall set of the biochemical analyses (Table 17). This table shows the values of the communalities obtained (i.e. the proportions of the variance of each parameter that can be related to the two

Table 17 Values of the communalities

	Factor 1	Factor 2
Cholic acid	0.86	0.81
Chenodeoxycholic acid	0.82	0.80
Lithocholic acid	0.66	0.66
SGOT	0.56	0.94
SGPT	0.49	0.94
Alkaline phosphatases	0.44	0.50
γ-GT	0.54	0.66
Total bilirubin	0.70	0.69
Prothrombin time	-0.57	-0.35
Serum albumin	-0.80	-0.49
Serum γ-globulins	0.57	0.31

factors). The two factors accounted for more than 80% of the variability of primary serum bile acids and for more than 90% of the variability of the transaminase serum levels.

Alkaline phosphatases, prothrombin time and serum γ-globulins were the parameters less correlated with the two factors. SGOT and SGPT depended mostly on the first factor while albumin and prothrombin time on the second one.

Cholic and chenodeoxycholic acids cannot be considered as tests identifying a specific liver function, but they are the tests more highly correlated with both the principal factors.

Setchell: I'm very concerned about the enormous effort that seems to be going on into assessing the predictive value of conventional bile acid measurements for liver disease. I wonder whether perhaps our efforts ought to be directed to some of the more unusual bile acids and to investigating their potential in predicting liver disease. When bile acids are measured by gas chromatography–mass spectrometry in serum samples from a variety of patients with liver disease, you see a large variety of different bile acids; probably 40. For example hyocholic acid is a feature of the serum bile acid profile of many patients with cholestasis, but I have yet to find this bile acid in normal subjects. Perhaps one should be directing efforts towards developing more convenient methods for measuring compounds such as this.

Gentilini: Orlandi's data are particularly brilliant. They are well presented and statistically perfect. They are also based on a standard which can be used in a general population. In fasting conditions, I do not think we can add anything to the other tests, as the serum bile acids are less sensitive, and here I agree with Orlandi. However, I think they should be considered as a loading test or a dynamic test in postprandial state. If we accept this concept, the only valid parameters for comparison are the galactose test, indocianine values and BSP.

So, the postprandial test could be re-evaluated as a loading test. This, however, does not concern the general population, but, and again I am in agreement with Orlandi, should be taken into consideration as a secondary test.

Orlandi: My opinion is that the bile acid tolerance tests are no more useful than the fasting tests.

Gentilini: I do not agree, because you must look for a loading test in comparison with other loading tests which can be carried out in follow-up patients, for example every 6 months during treatment. In this sense, transaminases, γ-GT, protein and prothrombin time tell us absolutely nothing, so that perhaps a valid loading test could still be the postprandial test. The comparison should be made in treated patients over a period of time. This was the sense of Mazzanti's communication.

Barbara: We do not agree.

Hofmann: I think this is a fascinating discussion and I think that the work presented is the finest work that I have ever heard presented on this subject. I think everyone here has made a very worthwhile contribution. It seems to me we have three problems. One is the technical problem, and if people can confirm the work of Roda, we may at last have a method as simple as transaminase. The second problem we have is: can we reduce the variability of the fasting state level? Can we control intestinal motility? I do not know, but we must think about it. It doesn't matter for other tests, but it matters for this fasting state test and the clinical chemist wants a fasting state test. For the loading tests we have a problem to develop an internal standard which will correct for all of the dynamic variables and we have not done that.

Barbara: The evaluation of efficiency is useful, but only as a first step, as it assumes that all misclassification mistakes are of equal importance. However, in my opinion, we need to consider the clinical cost of misclassifications, because an incorrect allocation has important diagnostic, prognostic and therapeutic implications. To improve the probability of successful treatment we have to define the effectiveness and the utility of the test. A discussion on the effectiveness is beyond the scope of this workshop but a few comments on the utility are relevant. Dr Festi, please.

Festi: I would like only to summarize our experience about the problem of misclassification. If we arbitrarily divide mild liver diseases (MLD), such as diseases not requiring therapy and normal subjects, from CAH and C, where therapy could be necessary, we observe that the combination LFT plus SBA allowed the better use of medical treatment (8.5% of CAH and C classified as MLD versus 10.5% and

10% classified by LFT and SBA, respectively) and vice-versa avoided an unneeded treatment (15.7% of MLD classified as CAH or C versus 16.3% and 21.3% by LFT and SBA, respectively).

Barbara: In conclusion even if some encouraging data exist, it does not seem that serum bile acid determination is more useful than conventional liver function tests, neither in defining the stage of liver disease nor in following the response to treatment. According to us, however, liver function tests may also be insufficient; clinical grading is better. As far as SBA's usefulness, in the field of particular liver diseases, is concerned the data presented are, without doubt, useful but not decisive in the global definition of the usefulness of the test.

REFERENCES

Almè, B., Bremmelgaard, A., Sjovall, J., et al. (1977). Analysis of metabolic profiles of bile acids in urine using a lipophilic anionic exchange and computerized gas-liquid chromatography mass spectrometry, *J. Lipid Res.*, **18**, 339

Anwer, M. S. and Hegner, D. (1979). Study of cholic acid conjugation by isolated rat hepatocytes, *Hoppe-Seyler's Z. Physiol, Chem.*, **360**, 515

Dyfverman, A. and Sjovall, J. (1978). Liquid-gel extraction of bile acids. In Paumgartner, G., Stiehl, A. and Gerok, W. (eds). *Biological Effects of Bile Acids*, pp. 281–6. (Lancaster: MTP Press)

Forker, E. L. and Luxon B. A. (1981). Albumin helps mediate removal of taurocholate by rat liver. *J. Clin. Invest.*, **67**, 1517

Heubi, J. E., Balistreri, W. F. and Suchy, F. J. (1982). Bile salt metabolism in the first year of life. *J. Lab. Clin. Med.*, **100**, 127

Kaplowitz, N., Kok, E. and Javitt, N. B. (1974). Postprandial serum bile acid for the detection of hepatobiliary disease. *J. Am. Med. Assoc.*, **225**, 292

LaRusso, N. F., Hoffman, N. E., Korman, M. G., et al. (1978). Determinants of fasting and postprandial serum bile acid levels in healthy man. *Am. J. Dig. Dis.*, **23**, 385

Matern, S. and Gerok, W. (1979). Diagnostic value of serum bile acids. *Acta Hepato-gastroenterol.*, **26**, 185

Porter, H. P. and Saunders, D. R. (1971). Isolation of the aqueous phase of human intestinal content during the digestion of a fatty meal. *Gastroenterology*, **60**, 997

Setchell, K. D. R., Lawson, A. M., Blackstok, E. J., et al. (1982). Diurnal changes in serum unconjugated bile acids in normal man. *Gut*, **23**, 637

Setchell, K. D. R. and Matsui, A. (1983). Serum bile acid analysis. *Clin. Chim. Acta*, **127**.

Setchell, K. D. R. and Worthingston, J. A. (1982). A rapid method for the quantitative extraction of bile acids and their conjugates from serum using commercially available reverse phase octadecylsilane bonded silica cartridge. *Clin. Chim. Acta*, **125**, 135

Suchy, F. J., Balistreri, W. F., Heubi, J. E., et al. (1981). Physiologic cholestasis: elevations of the primary serum bile acid concentration in normal infants. *Gastroenterology*, **80**, 1037

van Berge Henegouwen, G. P. and Hofmann, A. F. (1978). Nocturnal gallbladder storage and emptying in gallstone patients and healthy subjects. *Gastroenterology*, **75**, 879

Vlahcevic, Z. R., Miller, J. R., Farrar, J. P., *et al.* (1971). Kinetics and pool size of primary bile acids in man. *Gastroenterology*, **61**, 85

Watkins, J. B., Ingall, D., Szczepanik, P. A., *et al.* (1973). Bile salt metabolism in the newborn. Measurement of pool size and synthesis by stable isotope technic. *N. Engl. J. Med.*, **288**, 431

THE PATHOPHYSIOLOGY
OF THE
ENTEROHEPATIC CIRCULATION
OF BILE ACIDS

Hofmann: This workshop will be different from the other session that we have had in this meeting, as we are going to talk about what we do not understand, rather than what we do understand.

The first topic will be physicochemical studies related to bile acids and biliary lipid secretion. There will be four presentations dealing with rather theoretical topics; then, to balance the programme, there will be three brief reports dealing with clinical studies. The second part of the programme will be concerned with bile acid metabolism, cholesterol metabolism, and hepatic lysosomes. The next topic will be hepatic bile acid transport. There will then be several brief presentations of miscellaneous topics.

Dr Aldo Roda will begin our session by presenting his recent studies on the relationship between bile salt structure and micellar aggregation.

Roda: I would like to present new data based on studies carried out at the University of California in San Diego in the Department of Medicine, Division of Gastroenterology. The experiments were carried out in collaboration with our Chairman, Dr Alan F. Hofmann, and with Dr Carol J. Mysels, who is an international authority on micelles.

Let me begin with a very short introduction to the problem of bile salt association in water. Bile salts are considered detergent-like molecules, but they differ from the common ionic detergent in two respects. Typical ionic detergents contain a charged head group connected to a flexible aliphatic hydrophobic chain. In solution, they pack into large aggregates called micelles. Bile salts, on the other hand, have a structure in which the distinction between the polar and the non-polar part of the molecule is not so clear-cut. There is a rigid body with a hydrophobic face and a hydrophilic face. The side-chain is like that of typical ionic detergents in possessing a very strongly charged polar group at the end, but the length of the side-chain is much shorter. In solution, bile salts form small aggregates, and their association is more gradual – first dimers, then trimers, then oligomers.

For that reason, the number and the position of the hydroxy groups in the steroid nucleus of the bile salt and the structure of the side-chain play a key role in the self-association of these molecules in water. To date there have been few studies on the effect of bile salt structure on their aggregation. There have been studies related to the most common bile salts, such as chenodeoxycholate and cholate. Such studies have not provided a great insight into structure–aggregation relationships, since in the common bile salts the hydroxy groups are invariably in the alpha orientation and the side-chain is C_5 in length.

Therefore, we decided to carry out a systematic study of as many bile salts and bile salt analogues as we could obtain, believing that the study of compounds with considerable variation in substituent orientation on side-chain structure might provide additional insight into the relationship between structure and self-association water.

To do that we developed a new method to measure the aggregation of molecules in solution. The method is an improved maximum bubble pressure method. The principle of the method, which is not especially difficult, is as follows. When air is blown out of a capillary tube immersed in a liquid, a bubble is formed. The pressure in the bubble is maximal when the bubble is of minimum size, and that occurs when the diameter of the bubble is equal to the diameter of the tube. The pressure in the bubble can be recorded continuously and related to the surface tension in the solution. The bubble pressure can be recorded for different concentrations of bile salts which gives data permitting one to calculate the traditional surface tension–concentration curve.

For bile salts or any typical detergent, one obtains a curve with two slopes when one plots the surface tension against the logarithm of the concentration. The first slope, which is recorded at a low concentration of bile salt, indicates the surface acitivity of monomeric molecules. There is a change in the slope of the curve as self-association occurs in water. This slope is caused by a decrease in the rate at which the monomeric concentration increases. Since with bile salts this change occurs over a range of concentrations, we proposed a new name for this concentration region, namely 'uncritical'. Further, since the association of bile salts is gradual, we have termed the aggregates 'multimers' rather than monomers. Accordingly, the aim of this work was to study the relationship between bile salt structure and the concentration range over which association occurs, which we have termed an 'uncritical multimer concentration'. To validate the maximum bubble pressure method, we compared it against a completely independent method – the conventional dye solubilization procedure.

Altogether, 50 bile salts analogues were studied. The only monohydroxy bile salt that was soluble at room temperature was a 7-beta hydroxy bile salt. All the possible combinations of 3,7 and 3,12 dihydroxy bile salts were studied. A number of beta hydroxy epimers of trihydroxy bile salts were studied, as well as hydroxy oxo bile acids and peroxo bile acids, such as dehydrocholate.

In addition we studied the effect of side-chain amidation, i.e. conjugation with glycine or taurine on the UMC. We also determined the UMC of a zwitterionic bile salt, and of a non-ionic bile salt having a disaccharide side-chain. Finally, we studied the effect of side-chain length by comparing the aggregation of nor and bis-nor bile salts with their respective C_{24} homologues.

The correlation between the UMC data obtained by dye solubilization and by surface tension was excellent. The excellent agreement over a wide range of UMC values suggested that the two methods are valid for the measurement of the UMC in water and 0.15 mol/l sodium chloride.

As the side-chain was shortened the UMC increased exponentially. A plot of the log of UMC versus the number of carbons in the side-chain gave a straight line. A similar effect of chain length on the CMC of typical ionic detergents has been well established.

In general when an alpha hydroxy group was replaced by a beta hydroxy group, the UMC increased. However, in the 3,7 and 3,12 dihydroxy bile salts, the UMC of the di-beta hydroxy compounds were anomalously low. To rationalize this anomaly we examined molecular methods and photographed them. These experiments suggested that the UMC was related to the area of the continuous hydrophobic side of the molecule. The changing of an alpha to a beta hydroxy group decreased the hydrophobic region and increased the UMC value. However, with the di-beta hydroxy bile salts, the alpha side of the molecule, which is usually hydrophilic, now becomes hydrophobic; the beta side, which is usually hydrophobic, now becomes hydrophilic. With the tri-beta hydroxy bile salt, both sides of the molecule are hydrophilic, and although the UMC is still slightly lower than anticipated, it is still quite high.

Carey: It took our research group nearly 2 years to study one bile salt, and you have studied 50 bile salts in 1 year. However, let me make a comment. When one uses surface tension to measure the CMC, one uses the change in surface properties to provide an indication of what is happening in the bulk phase. Unless the surface is in equilibrium with the bulk phase, surface properties will not be a valid indicator of bulk events. I believe you have not demonstrated unequivocally that you have obtained true equilibrium with the maximum bubble pressure method. In fact, the maximum bubble pressure method is well known not to provide a valid indication of equilibrium surface tension. My question is this. What justifies you in changing the conventional critical micellar concentration to the uncritical multimer concentration? What the CMC is depends on the bile salt and on the condition.

Roda: I agree. In fact, we used not only the maximum bubble pressure method and dye solubilization to measure the UMC, but in addition we used conductivity and spectral shifts. With all of these methods the aggregation appears to occur over a concentration range so that there really is no well-defined CMC, as one observes with a typical ionic detergent such as sodium dodecyl sulphate.

Carey: Do you not think that multimer formation occurs over quite a narrow concentration range for sodium taurodeoxycholate in 0.15 mol/l sodium?

Dowling: Our next speaker is Dr Carey.

Carey: I am going to present in some detail Dr Salvioli's work which he performed during an extended visit to our laboratory in Boston. For some time now, we have been interested in developing a rational model for understanding how bile salts can remove large quantities of membrane lipids as they flux through the liver cell. To look at this question we designed a simple experimental model which, we believe, may provide base-line information on bile salt detergency.

  We use millipore filters of ~ 3 μm pore size, wash them in benzene to remove contaminating hydrocarbons and then soak them in a lipid–benzene solution. Such a solution can contain any membrane lipid or lipid mixture that one desires but in most of our experiments we employed cholesterol and egg yolk lecithin in a molar ratio of 0.3. The organic solvent was then evaporated and the membranes were soaked in Tris buffer (pH 7.4) containing physiological concentrations of sodium chloride. With these procedures cholesterol–lecithin mixtures had deposited in the pores of the millipore membranes and had swelled to form artificial membranes as demonstrated by electron microscopy.

  We then mounted the filter-membranes in a modified Swinney apparatus and perfused bile salt solutions through them at a known rate. The effluents were collected every 10 min for 90 min and cholesterol–lecithin concentrations were measured. We perfused all the common and several uncommon taurine conjugated bile salts in concentrations ranging from 0.25 to 8 mmol/l. During each perfusion there was a first-order decrease in the eluted concentrations of both cholesterol and lecithin as functions of time. For comparable perfusing concentrations the most hydrophilic bile salts (tauroursodeoxycholate and taurohyodeoxycholate) removed much less lipid than the most hydrophobic bile salts (taurodeoxycholate and taurochenodeoxycholate).

  When all these data were summed over time and plotted as elution rates versus bile salt concentration, the two most hydrophobic bile salts gave a similar pattern, that of a rectangular hyperbola convex upwards. The curves for the two most hydrophilic bile salts were shaped in the opposite direction. Taurocholate, a bile salt of inter-mediate hydrophilicity, removed very little lecithin or cholesterol up to a concentration of 2 mmol/l. Then between 2 and 3 mmol/l, i.e. in the vicinity of the CMC, a sharp increase occurred and between 3 and 8 mmol/l only a slight further increase was observed.

The cholesterol to lecithin ratios in the effluents were then plotted against the bile salt concentration perfused. In the case of tauro-cholate, taurochenodeoxycholate and taurodeoxycholate there was no significant change in the cholesterol–lecithin ratio compared with that in the model membranes. However, with tauroursodeoxy-cholate and taurohyodeoxycholate there was a 50% decrease in the cholesterol–lecithin ratio in the effluents compared with that in the artificial membranes.

The average lipid outputs for a physiological mixture of tauro-cholate, taurochenodeoxycholate and taurodeoxycholate (40 : 40 : 20) were then plotted versus bile salt output. The curves were remarkably reminiscent of that found *in vivo* in man and other animals, in that the amount of lecithin was greater than the amount of cholesterol secreted and in both cases the curvilinear relationships tended to plateau at high bile salt outputs. Thus we have described an apparatus that is capable of making bile in the laboratory. This similarity of our *in vitro* results to that of *in vivo* systems during bile secretion suggests that bile salt detergency is physiologically relevant.

Hofmann: Might I begin by asking whether you have studied glycine conjugates?

Carey: We get a rather similar pattern provided they are completely ionized. All of the glycine conjugates, particularly glycoursodeoxy-cholate, only become completely ionized at pH 9 and above. As you decrease the pH there is a profound pH-dependent decrease in lipid secretion. Dr Salvioli may like to make another comment on that.

Salvioli: Glycoursodeoxycholate and glycoursodeoxycholate were perfused at a 4 mmol/l concentration, but the induced secretion of lipids in the effluent was higher when the pH of the solution was 9 instead of 7. However, we think that the use of glycine conjugates of pH 9 is hazardous, because pH 9 may induce hydrolysis of the lecithin. That is why we have used taurine conjugates which are fully ionized at a more physiological and less dangerous pH.

Carey: Yes, but there is a more important point. When one employs a pH just above the precipitation pH, the micelles are saturated with their own acid species. As Salvioli said, this has an important influence on lipid binding. Other studies along these lines are in progress.

Dowling: I think these data are absolutely fascinating. The obvious question is: how do the results obtained with this model relate to transport of bile acids through the canalicular membrane and to the transport of lipids into bile? You have shown diminishing lipid 'secretion' with time. Is there enough lipid in the artificial membrane to ensure that the progressive leaching of the lipid from the membrane with a resultant dimininishing 'secretion', is not simply due to reduction in the amount of substrate available?

Carey: I pointed out that when high bile salt concentrations were perfused there was a first-order decrease in lipid outputs. So we were decreasing the pool size within the membranes. However, using very slow perfusion rates, increases in the number of membranes or low bile salt concentrations, we were able to obtain a pseudo-steady state. The experiments we are planning now involve terminating such experiments every 10 min, extracting the lecithin and cholesterol, and measuring the amounts remaining. By knowing the pool at 10 min intervals we should be able to correct the curves to obtain zero-order kinetics.

Dowling: There is enough substrate remaining?

Carey: Oh yes, we remove only between about 5% to a maximum of 50% of total lipids. This depends on the bile salt species, its concentration and the perfusion time.

Dowling: Fine. My second question relates to the bile acid concentrations you used since this presumes that we might actually approach a millimolar bile acid concentration within the liver cell or traversing the membrane. I have just forgotten the bile acid concentrations which you used?

Carey: Well, we used bile salt concentrations which varied between 0.25 mmol/l, that is 250 μmol/l, and 8 mmol/l. The highest concentration of bile salts that has been reported to be in the liver cell is about

300 μmol/l. However, nobody knows what concentrations are in the endoplasmic reticulum, in or around the canalicular membranes or in the canalicular lumen.

Dowling: That is precisely the point. There is the idea that you have got to build up a micellar concentration, whether you call it CMC or UMC, on the *outer* aspect of the canalicular membrane, thereby selectively leaching out lipids only from the outer half of the membrane.

Carey: You obviously have heard of phospholipid transporting proteins in the liver. Bile salts are phospholipid- and cholesterol-transporting lipids, and we have shown here that they can transport lipids even below the CMCs of the pure materials. We really do not understand what the intermicellar concentration is in the presence of lots of lipids. It is probably very low. However, at these low bile salt concentrations, bile salts can form other structures with membrane lipids such as vesicles. So bile salts might be involved in transporting lipids as vesicles from the endoplasmic reticulum, i.e. the site of synthesis to the canalicular membrane, the site of secretion. I strongly doubt that mixed micelles are present within liver cells.

Dowling: This supposes, then, that you have lipid transport at bile acid concentrations lower than the CMC?

Carey: Yes, I think so.

Dowling: Now, that is pre-micellar association, is that right?

Carey: I do not know what you mean.

Dowling: Dr Roda and I have agreed to let you call this phenomenon 'secretion' if you will let us continue to talk about the CMC! But, to be serious, I would like to point out that there is a striking difference between your data, where you compare taurocheno and taurourso, with the data of Gilmore *et al.* (1982) in the dog, where taurourso and taurocheno were really rather similar. Both these bile acids pulled out more lecithin and more cholesterol than did taurocholate. So there are major differences between the animal findings and your *in vitro* results.

Carey: Well, I am not sure. It depends on your point of view. The detergent effects may be the same but metabolic effects may alter the final *in vivo* results in the direction you mention.

Dowling: I think if we could interpret the results of your *in vitro* system, it would help us to understand the *in vivo* system. So I am all for this.

Angelico: What kind of lecithin did you use? Was it a mixture of different lecithins? And what was the composition of the lecithin which was eluted?

Carey: You have asked a very important question. Dr Angelico is asking indirectly why bile salts couple specific phospholipids species such as lecithin and within that species why the 16:0, 18:1 and 16:0, 18:2 fatty acid subclasses. As you know well, egg lecithin is very similar to biliary lecithin so we would not have expected any big change. We are tackling this problem with mixtures of hepatic lecithins.

Fromm: I think your system is very attractive. The question is, if you study the same bile acid in terms of effect on biliary lecithin secretion, would it explain the difference in animal species? What I am driving at is, is induced biliary lipid secretion explicable solely by physical–chemical mechanisms, or are there other factors? Perhaps we must compare the *in vitro* model with the effects of bile acids on lecithin secretion in a variety of species.

Carey: Yes, the question you are asking is: is the coupling not only with lecithin, but is the specific subclass of lecithin purely physical–chemical. I do not know if it is or is not. From what I have been able to learn, there is nothing special about the lecithin in bile, either at monolayers or in bulk, that makes it especially different physically or chemically. But there may be reasons downstream that make this subspecies important, especially in terms of its role in forming the surface coat of chylomicrons.

Hofmann: The next speaker is Dr Graham, who is working with Dr Northfield, and who has been carrying out similar studies with isolated bile canalicular membranes.

Graham: I hope to address myself to the point which Professor Dowling made about the possibility of bile acids actually removing lipids from the bile canalicular membrane once they get into the canaliculus. Like Dr Carey we, at St George's Hospital Medical School, in association with Dr Northfield, are working on a model system to try and explain the effect of bile acid secretion on the appearance of lipids in the bile. In Dr Carey's elegant model he is looking more at the transfer of bile acid molecules across the membrane. We are one stage further on. We are trying to use a model to look at the removal of lipid from the membrane once the bile acids are in the canaliculus.

We are using the hamster as a human model and we have isolated the bile canalicular membrane from hamster liver. To identify the source of our membrane preparations we had used enzyme analysis. It is well established that in the bile canalicular membrane the levels of 5'-nucleotidase, alkaline phosphodiesterase and beta-naphthyl-amidase, are much higher than in any other part of the hepatocyte plasma membrane.

Table 1   Enzyme analysis of membrane fractions

Enzyme	BCM*	Contiguous
5'-nucleotidase	47.44	5.22
Alkaline phosphodiesterase	48.57	7.53
β-naphthylamidase	6.41	0.89
Glucagon-stimulated adenylate cyclase	0.00	0.80

*BCM = Bile canalicular membrane
All enzyme activities are expressed as μmol of substrate utilized h^{-1} mg protein^{-1}

The method which we use enables us to isolate simultaneously the bile canalicular membrane and the contiguous membrane. Table 1 shows that the bile canalicular membrane does have a significant enrichment in these enzymes over the contiguous membrane. An enzyme which has been shown to be absent in the bile canalicular membrane is the glucagon-stimulated adenylate cyclase, which is heavily enriched in the sinusoidal membrane and to some extent also in the contiguous membrane. This enzyme is undetectable in our bile canalicular membrane preparation.

Furthermore this membrane, as it is isolated, exists in the form of small vesicles. Panel A in Fig. 1 shows a freeze-fracture electron micro-graph of the fraction: the profile of these vesicles is quite clear; whilst the contiguous membranes form large sheets, as shown on Panel B.

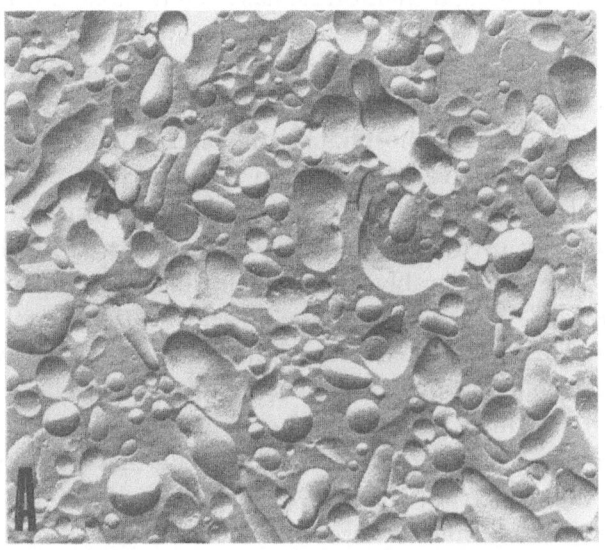

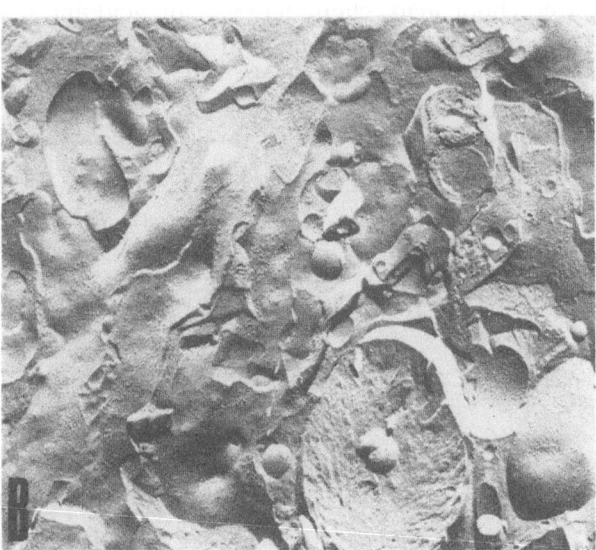

Figure 1 Freeze-fracture electron micrographs of hamster liver membrane fractions. Panel A: vesicles of bile canalicular membrane; panel B: sheets of contiguous membrane

The bile canalicular membrane has been incubated with bile acids and the lipids they leach out have been analysed. The incubations were originally carried out in phosphate buffered saline; this has been changed to Hepes-buffered saline in recent experiments to eliminate any interference from phosphate in the phospholipid analysis. In our earlier experiments each incubation contained 180 g of membrane protein/ml, and bile salts at concentration of between 1 and 4 mmol/l were routinely used, although in our first experiment the concentrations were considerably higher than that. The membranes were incubated at 37 °C for 5 min in the presence of the bile salts and then transferred to 4 °C and centrifuged: the membrane pellet was washed once in ice-cold phosphate buffered saline or Hepes buffered saline, and then the final pellet and the first supernatant analysed for cholesterol and phospholipid. In all the data that I shall present we have used taurine conjugates of the bile acids.

Although some contention exists about the value of the CMC of these bile acids, most workers agree that it is below 32 mmol/l and probably in the range 1–4 mmol/l. In the first series of experiments we compared cholic acid, chenodeoxycholic acid and dehydrocholic acid at 32 mmol/l. Dehydrocholic acid is not a micelle-forming bile acid even at this high concentration.

Table 2 Solubilization of lipids from bile canalicular membrane by bile acids at 32 mmol/l concentration

	Percentage lipid solubilized	
Bile acid	Phospholipid	Cholesterol
Cholic	90	95
Chenodeoxycholic	98	95
Dehydrocholic	0	0

Table 2 shows that both cholic acid and chenodeoxycholic acid totally solubilized the membrane: virtually all the phospholipid was removed and all the cholesterol; whereas dehydrocholate removed absolutely no cholesterol or phospholipid from the membrane whatsoever. Thus it appears that in this particular *in vitro* system, micelle formation is very important for the solubilization of membrane lipid.

In the next series of experiments we compared cholic acid and chenodeoxycholic acid at the lower concentrations previously mentioned, i.e. between 1 and 4 mmol/l. From Fig. 2 it is clear that

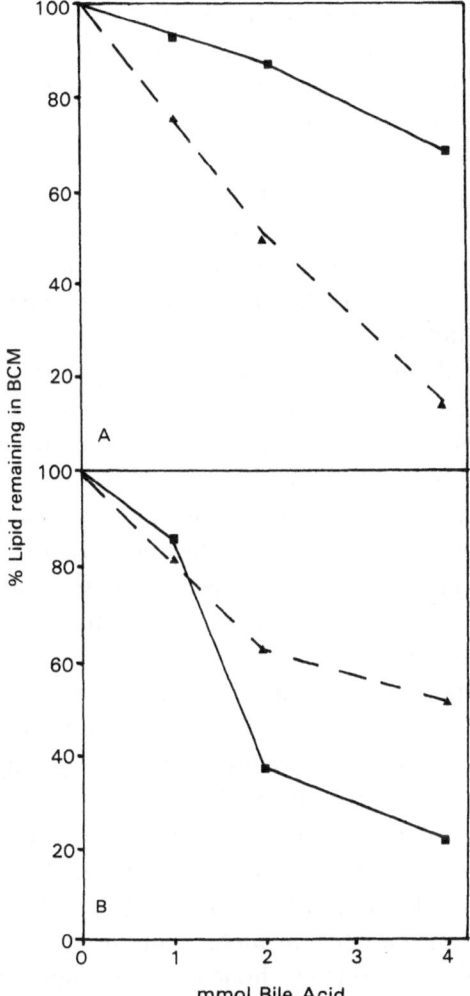

Figure 2 Solubilization of lipid from hamster bile canalicular membrane (BCM) by cholic acid (panel A); chenodeoxycholic acid (panel B). The incubations contained 0.18 mg BCM protein/ml. —■—■— phospholipid; — ▲ — ▲ — cholesterol

chenodeoxycholic acid was far more effective in extracting phospholipid than cholesterol: on the other hand cholic acid was far more effective at removing cholesterol than phospholipid.

In these particular experiments the membrane protein concentration was 0.18 mg/ml: even though the freeze-fracture electron micrographs showed that the vesicles are still intact, at this level of bile canalicular membrane, approximately 60% of the total protein was removed at a bile acid concentration of 4 mmol/l.

In the next series of experiments the amount of bile canalicular membrane was increased to 0.4 mg protein/ml. Under these conditions, even at a 4 mmol/l concentration of bile acid, less than 10% of the membrane protein was removed during incubation. Moreover, using these higher concentrations of membrane the importance of micelle formation is much more evident. At low concentrations of bile acid (below 1 mmol/l) deoxycholate, chenodeoxycholate and ursodeoxycholate (Fig. 3) solubilize little or no cholesterol or phospholipid from the membrane. If the critical micellar concentration for both chenodeoxycholate and deoxycholate is between 1 and 2 mmol/l, it appears that above this level there is a significant solubilization of both cholesterol and phospholipid. But while deoxycholate solubilizes both cholesterol and phospholipid, virtually simultaneously, Fig. 3 shows that chenodeoxycholic acid starts to remove phospholipid from the membrane at a much lower concentration than that required to start removing cholesterol from the membrane. This difference is completely reproducible. Ursodeoxycholate acid only begins to remove both the cholesterol and phospholipid at around 4 mmol/l under these *in vitro* conditions.

Although the effect of chenodeoxycholic acid on lipid solubilization was similar at both the low and high membrane protein concentrations, i.e. it showed a preference for phospholipid removal over cholesterol removal; the effect of cholic acid was very dependent on the membrane concentration. At low concentrations of membrane, cholic acid solubilized a lot of cholesterol and phospholipid at low concentrations (1–2 mmol/l) of bile acid (Fig. 2) – at the higher concentration of bile canalicular membrane the pattern of solubilization resembled that of ursodeoxycholic acid, i.e. significant solubilization only occurred around 4 mmol/l concentration.

Von Bergman: Have you looked at what kind of phospholipids and cholesterol you have removed from your membranes?

Graham: No, we are obviously keen to do this and we are about to embark on a series of experiments in which we are going to look at the species of phospholipids which are removed using high-performance liquid chromatography.

Carey: I am concerned about one kind of key issue here and that is: are the bile salts in nature bathing the outer leaflet of the canalicular

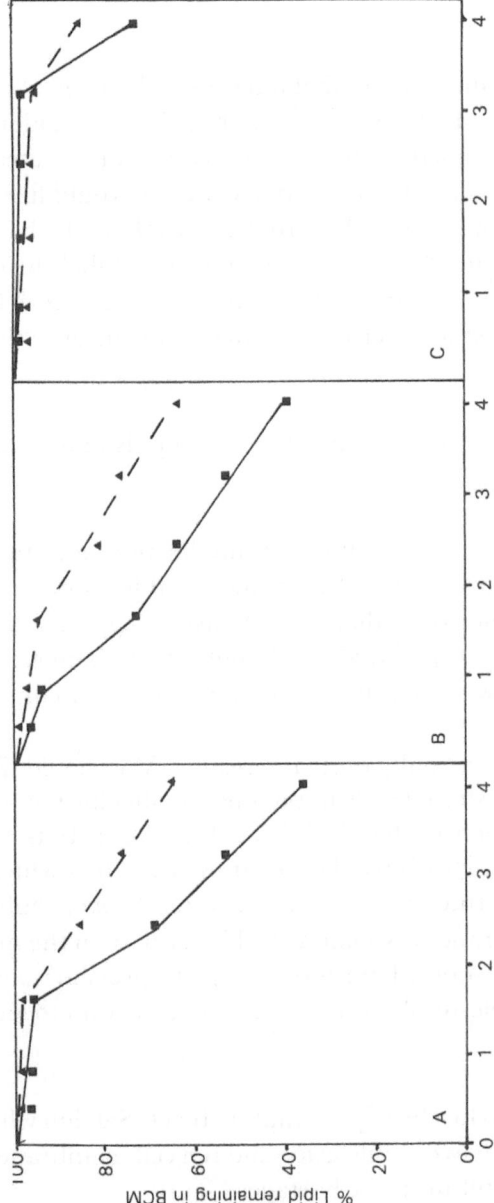

Figure 3 Solubilization of lipid from hamster bile canalicular membrane (BCM) by deoxycholic acid (panel A); chenodeoxycholic acid (panel B); ursodeoxycholic acid (panel C). The incubations contained 0.4 mg BCM protein/ml. ——■—— phospholipid; —▲——▲— cholesterol

membrane long enough to do what you have just shown? I mean, I know when we inject [^{14}C]taurocholate we can measure it way downstream, miles downstream in 10 sec. What kind of time frame are we talking about?

Graham: I really cannot answer that question. All the incubations were done over a period of 5 min and although we could reduce the incubation time to maybe a minute or a couple of minutes, it makes things practically very difficult to do. What we would like to do is to try and address ourselves to this problem by taking the hamsters and injecting them with [^{14}C]mevalonate and ^{32}P to label the cholesterol and the phospholipid prior to doing this analysis; then I think we might be able to get a better idea of what happens over shorter time periods.

Carey: At the same time we will extract the lipids and pump the bile salts through them.

Balistrieri: One point that might be of implication, and that is if you looked at the fluidity of the membranes in this context. The point being that in the newborn there is a change in apparent lipid microviscosity, as the phospholipids and cholesterol changes. This may have, as you know, a significant functional implication.

Graham: Yes, that is actually quite interesting. We should like to have a look at the cholesterol levels in the bile canalicular membrane and how this may influence what the bile acids take out. In this last series of experiments which I have described the hamsters which we used were quite obese. Interestingly, the cholesterol : phospholipid molar ratio in the membrane was some 20 % higher than in the membranes prepared from non-obese hamsters used in the previous experiments. So I think that cholesterol status is something we want to look at quite closely.

Dowling: We now go to a brief presentation by Dr Salvioli who will look at the interaction between bile acids and red cell membranes. It looks as if this field is still in its early stages.

Salvioli: My presentation deals with the effects of bile salts (tauroconjugates) on living membranes (erythrocytes). It is well recognized that the modifications of the lipid content of red blood cell (RBC) membranes result in haemolysis occurring either after extensive depletion of cholesterol (C) or after accumulation of lecithin (Lec); in general when fluidity of the membranes is reduced a rapid haemolysis occurs. In human RBC membranes sphingomyelin (SM) and lecithin (zwitterionic phospholipids, PL) are predominantly located in the outer layer, whereas phosphatidylserine and phosphatidylethanolamine are in the inner half. In ruminants (cow) the outer layer contains above all SM which is less fluid than Lec owing to: (1) the high saturated fatty acid content, and (2) the *trans*-double-bond in the sphingosine chain (able to increase the rigidity of the molecule).

We studied the haemolytic effect and the solubilization of the membranes observed when bovine and human RBC membranes are incubated with isotonic solutions of tauroconjugates, namely taurodeoxycholate (TDC), taurochenodeoxycholate (TCDC), taurocholate (TC) and tauroursocholate (TUDC) having a decreasing hydrophobicity. Washed RBC of man and cow are incubated at 37 °C for 45 min suspended in a medium represented by isotonic Tris buffer 5 mmol/l, pH 7.4, containing or not containing different concentrations (0.27–8 mmol/l) of tauroconjugates; the final Ht was constant. The events of haemolysis are followed by interference contrast microscopy; after centrifugation at 15,000 rpm: (a) the percentage of haemolysis, and (b) the amount of lipids (C and PL) solubilized are determined in the supernatant. The extent of haemolysis was higher with TDC > TCDC > TUDC > TC and when human erythrocytes are incubated. Only the most hydrophobic tauroconjugates (TDC and TCDC) promote haemolysis at 0.5–2 mmol/l, below their CMC, and solubilize membrane lipids with C/PL molar ratio values increasing with bile salt concentrations. TCD and TCDC induce echinocyte formation below their CMC, On the contrary TC and TUDC induce echinocyte formation only at concentrations > 4 mmol/l; they are less lytic than TDC and TCDC and C/PL ratio of solubilized lipids decreases with high concentrations of TUDC; when human RBC are incubated, C/PL molar ratio in the solubilized lipids is higher with respect to bovine RBC. When bile salts are added with Lec, the haemolytic effect is lower; it seems that RBC membrane lipid composition affects the amount of lipids removed by bile salts and that the most hydrophilic (TC and TUDC) are less lytic on erythrocytes.

Balistrieri: How does your work relate to the old idea of Cooper that lithocholate is responsible for spur cell formation in liver disease? Do you think that elevated levels of other serum bile acids might cause this abnormality in liver disease?

Salvioli: The concentration of serum bile acids during spur cell anaemia is not very high. Spur cell formation is due to the increase of cholesterol with respect to phospholipids in the red cell membrane. I think that bile acids are not directly responsible for the formation of irregular contour of erythrocytes.

Hofmann: Why do bile acids cause haemolysis?

Salvioli: I do not know exactly; it is an isotonic haemolysis.

Hofmann: Why do bile salts induce haemolysis?

Salvioli: Probably they increase the RBC membrane permeability or they chop up the membrane lipid components of the membrane and above all the outer layer components (Lec and SM).

Hofmann: Do you think that phospholipid solubilization is necessary to produce haemolysis?

Salvioli: I think so.

Hofmann: I wonder. Lithocholate is very haemolytic, but should be a very bad solubilizer. Could it be an exception to your statement?

Salvioli: Probably lithocholate has another action: it can enter the membranes intercalating their components.

Dowling: Your descriptions of RCM distortion are very similar to those seen in some forms of chronic liver disease, where the molar ratio of cholesterol : cholesterol ester in the membrane is altered and this results in distortion of the red cell. Obviously if we are thinking of extrapolating from these results to lipid transport across the bile canalicular membrane into bile, we are talking about free cholesterol. Do you know whether cholesterol ester or free cholesterol or both were affected in this system?

Graham: I must say that I think it is unlikely that there is any significant amount of cholesterol ester in any plasma membrane.

Hofmann: We must depart from these fascinating *in vitro* studies which seem to raise more questions than answers. We are going to have three brief reports of clinical studies.

Sama: We know that chronic administration of chenodeoxycholic and ursodeoxycholic acids decreases cholesterol secretion and dissolves cholesterol gallstones, but the mechanisms involved are still unclear. The mechanisms that might account for the diminished hepatic cholesterol secretion induced by these two lithocholic bile acids are:

(a) a decreased hepatic synthesis of cholesterol;
(b) a diminished intestinal absorption of cholesterol; or
(c) a decreased bile acid–cholesterol secretory coupling by the liver.

We investigated the effect of acute bile acid administration on biliary lipid secretion in eight healthy subjects by means of a perfusion technique (Sama *et al.*, 1982). We measured bile acid, cholesterol and phospholipid outputs before, during and after replacing the bile acid pool with cholic, cheno or ursodeoxycholic acids. We substituted the endogenous bile acid pool by more than 75% with each of the three bile acids and we obtained the following results:

(a) As far as bile acid–cholesterol secretory coupling is concerned we found significantly less cholesterol secreted per mole of bile acid after pool replacement with urso ($p = 0.05$), than after cheno or cholic acid infusion.
(b) Although acute replacement with chenodeoxycholic acid did not significantly alter the secretory coupling of lecithin to bile acid, replacement with either ursodeoxycholic or cholic acid reduced ($p = 0.05$) the amount of lecithin secreted per mole of bile acid.

The main finding of this study was that acute replacement of endogenous bile acid pool with chenodeoxycholic, ursodeoxycholic or cholic acid in healthy subjects, alters the hepatic secretion of cholesterol and phospholipid in a consistent fashion.

We proposed that the major mechanism whereby acute bile acid pool replacement alters biliary lipid secretion is modulation of the secretory coupling of bile acids to cholesterol and phospholipid.

Mazzella: Production of cholesterol supersaturated bile may be due, in obese subjects, to increased cholesterol secretion rate, and in normal-weight subjects with gallstones, to decreased secretion of bile acids. Considering their different behaviours, four obese (131% ideal weight) and four non-obese (94% ideal weight) subjects with cholesterol gallstones in functioning gallbladder, were chosen, and biliary lipid secretion rates were studied before and after chronic administration (1 month in cross-over for each group) of chenodeoxycholic acid (CDCA) ($12.5\,\mathrm{mg\,kg^{-1}\,day^{-1}}$) and ursodeoxycholic acid (UDCA) ($7.5\,\mathrm{mg\,kg^{-1}\,day^{-1}}$) in order to evaluate the mechanism by which they induce the formation of cholesterol undersaturated bile.

Both bile acids induced a decrease in cholesterol secretion in both groups: in obese patients, CDCA from 85 ± 32 mg/h to 62 ± 15 mg/h ($p < 0.05$) and UDCA from 85 ± 32 mg/h to 54 ± 11 mg/h ($p < 0.05$); in normal-weight subjects, CDCA from 36 ± 7 mg/h to 31 ± 11 mg/h, and UDCA from 36 ± 7 mg/h to 26.5 ± 6.5 mg/h ($p < 0.005$). No effects were observed on bile acid and phospholipid secretion rates.

Finally to give a preliminary report on biliary secretion with UDCA and tauroursodeoxycholic acid (TUDCA) in one obese and non-obese subject, it may be observed that TUDCA induced a further decrease in cholesterol secretion rate over UDCA without affecting other biliary lipid secretion rate.

Hofmann: Might I note that these experiments are quite different from those reported by Dr Sama. She reported changes in biliary lipid secretion associated with acute replacement of the bile acid pool, whereas Dr Mazzella's results described changes occurring after 1 month of bile acid therapy. Could I ask Dr Mazzella if he actually measured the proportion of biliary bile acids which became composed of tauroursodeoxycholate?

Mazzella: We have not completely defined the pattern of biliary bile acids, but we did observe that about 50% of the bile acids were conjugated with taurine.

Hofmann: In fact, that means the mole fraction of bile acids conjugated with glycine has diminished from only 75% to 50%.

Carulli: These data concern the effect on biliary lipid secretion of acute duodenal infusion of CA and CDCA.

The study was carried out on three T-tube patients who received the two bile acids at 3-day intervals. The experiment was divided into two periods. A pretreatment period of 5 h starting with the complete interruption of EHC, followed by a replacement period of 5 h during which the bile acid was infused at a rate of 1 g/h. Bile was collected hourly during the whole study and analysed for lipid content.

Table 3 Relationship between bile acid, cholesterol and phospholipid biliary secretion

Output/mol BA	Pretreatment	CDCA	CA
Cholesterol	0.196*	0.078	0.050
Phospholipid	0.341	0.177	0.129

*The figures refer to the values of the slopes of the regression lines

Table 3 shows the slope values of the curves relating bile acid to cholesterol and phospholipid secretion. They suggest that CDCA infusion stimulates a bile lipid secretion greater than that obtained with CA infusion. Preliminary data on UDCA infusion show that with this bile acid bile lipid secretion is the lowest. With DCA infusion, at the dose employed, we observed signs of cholestasis.

Hofmann: Dr Reno Vlahcevic has told me in a personal communication that they also observed a cholestatic effect when deoxycholic acid was given to a patient with a bile fistula.

Carey: I would like to suggest that there is considerable intellectual unity in these diverse presentations. It seems to me that ursodeoxycholate, whether given acutely or chronically, is expressing the same detergent properties which it displays in our model system. I would suggest to Dr Carulli that his experimental results may be influenced by the creation of an acute taurine deficiency. We must not forget that the hydrophilicity of bile acids is determined, at least to some extent, by their mode of conjugation. Why not load the liver with taurine before or during your experiments?

Hofmann: Dr Carey makes a very important suggestion. However, I am not convinced there is total intellectual unity. The Swinney adapters, and the results in man agree; but results in animals, such as the hamster and dog, do not.

Von Bergmann: Our published results support Dr Carey's speculation. If you measure the glycine and taurine conjugates in patients with T-tubes after giving 1 g of chenodeoxycholic or cholic acid, you can show that the proportion conjugated with glycine increases from 75% to 95%. So there really is acute depletion of the taurine pool in the liver.

Dowling: The next section of the workshop deals with lipoproteins. Could I ask Dr Donald Small to tell us about the role of lipoproteins in the hepatic uptake of cholesterol and in bile acid formation?

Small: I have been asked on short notice to give a brief summary of the cholesterol balance across the liver and I would like to start with this rather crude cartoon (Fig. 4) which estimates the very approximate situation in a normal human. On the input side is lipoprotein uptake and *de novo* cholesterol synthesis and on the output side, metabolism of cholesterol to bile salt, secretion of lipoproteins (VLDL) and secretion of biliary cholesterol.

   Considering output from the liver, about 0.3 g of cholesterol are converted to bile salt a day. From the work of Bennion and Grundy

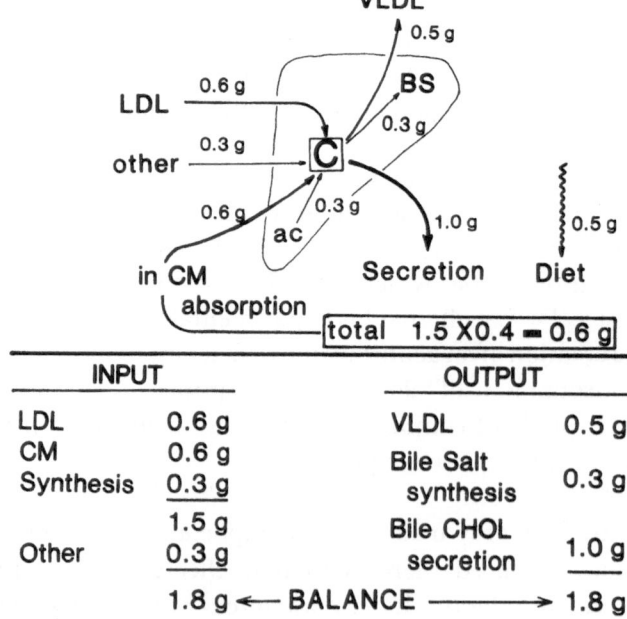

INPUT		OUTPUT	
LDL	0.6 g	VLDL	0.5 g
CM	0.6 g	Bile Salt	
Synthesis	0.3 g	synthesis	0.3 g
	1.5 g	Bile CHOL	
Other	0.3 g	secretion	1.0 g
	1.8 g ←	BALANCE →	1.8 g

Figure 4   Cholesterol balance across the liver

(1975) and others I estimate that about 0.5 g is secreted into very low density lipoprotein (VLDL) and enters the plasma. Finally, about 1 g of cholesterol is secreted into bile per day. Thus, the total output from the liver is about 1.8 g per day. These of course are very rough figures but will serve to illustrate some points.

Now consider the input side. Let us assume we have a very low egg diet and ingest 0.5 g of cholesterol. Also entering the intestine is the 1 g of endogenous cholesterol coming mainly from the biliary secretion, giving a total of 1.5 g entering the gut per day. If the coefficient of absorption is around 0.4 then about 0.6 g of the total 1½ g that goes into the intestine is reabsorbed. It is largely packaged in the form of chylomicrons and makes its way back into the liver as chylomicron remnants.

A very important experiment was carried out several years ago; it was shown that if you label LDL with sucrose you do not change its behaviour physically or its behaviour in relation to receptors. However, the sucrose taken up by cells remains in the cell and is not degraded. Thus, sucrose serves as a marker for LDL uptake by tissues. It was found that about half of injected labelled LDL ends up in the liver. Since we know that the overall turnover of LDL cholesterol is about 1.2 g a day we can estimate that about half of that (0.6 g) ends up in the liver. Finally, in the liver there is the *de novo* synthesis of about 0.3 g of cholesterol a day. That is about half the total body synthesis, the rest being made in other tissues. Thus, we estimate the input to the liver to be about 1.5 g, or about 0.3 g less than the output. That means another 0.3 g must get into the liver in some way to balance input with output.

Let us examine the mechanism by which cholesterol gets into the liver. A variety of receptors for specific apo-lipoproteins have been found on liver plasma membranes; these include the classical LDL receptor first described by Goldstein and Brown (1977) in fibroblast. This receptor is strongly regulated by the hepatocyte concentration of free cholesterol. Thus, when free cholesterol is depleted from the liver, for instance, by biliary fistula or cholestyramine treatment, the hepatic receptor is induced and appears in abundance in liver membranes. This receptor functions at a relatively low level of efficiency in humans, but it is probably responsible for the removal of approximately 6 g of LDL cholesterol per day from plasma into liver. This receptor may possibly be regulated in the same way by bile acids, since the recent United States National Cooperative Gallstone Study

(Albers *et al.*, 1982) showed that feeding chenodeoxycholic acid increased the plasma LDL levels significantly. This effect might be related to chenodeoxycholic acid blocking bile salt synthesis from cholesterol, thus increasing hepatocyte cholesterol and in turn turning off the LDL receptor, or it might be related to a direct effect of bile salt on the receptor.

It has also been shown that the LDL receptor is also quite capable of taking up the lipoprotein which contains apolipoprotein E or 'arginine-rich' apolipoprotein. Thus, lipoproteins in the plasma containing apolipoprotein E might be removed by the LDL receptor and the cholesterol in these lipoproteins delivered to the liver. The quantitative extent of this removal mechanism is not known.

A second receptor is also present in human and animal liver cells. The strongest evidence for such a receptor comes from the fact that patients with *LDL receptor deficiency* (homozygous familial hypercholesterolaemia) who have no receptors for LDL clear chylomicron remnants readily from the circulation. Thus, there is a chylomicron remnant receptor(s) distinct from the LDL receptor. The work of several investigators has produced evidence that this receptor recognizes apolipoprotein E (apoE). After secretion from the intestines chylomicrons adsorb apoliproprotein E as they circulate in the plasma. ApoE-rich chylomicron remnants are readily taken up by this receptor. The receptor might be called the 'apoE receptor', and should be distinguished from the apoLDL which is an apoB/E receptor. Further, this receptor does not appear to be tightly regulated by hepatic cholesterol content. To complicate things further it has been shown that intestinal apolipoprotein B (or the 'apoB-48' of Kane) may also be a ligand for a chylomicron receptor. Since intestinal apoB is secreted only on intestinal particles (specifically chylomicrons of intestinal VLDL) it is technologically appealing to consider this apolipoprotein as a ligand for hepatic uptake of dietary lipids.

Finally, some cholesterol which is synthesized in or delivered to peripheral tissue must be removed from tissue and delivered back to the liver. Since the discovery of cholesterol ester transport proteins in the rabbit, a large number of species, including man, have been found to have proteins capable of transferring cholesterol esters from cholesterol-rich lipoproteins such as HDL to triglyceride-rich lipoproteins. Thus, cholesterol which is removed from tissues by the HDL system and converted by lecithin cholesterol acyltransferase

(LCAT) to cholesterol ester may be transferred from high-density lipoproteins (major substrates for LCAT) to VLDL or chylomicrons, and thus some of the cholesterol from tissue may be transported back to the liver through LDL and chylomicron remnants. Furthermore, apoE containing HDL can be taken up by either the LDL receptor or the apoE receptor and returned to the liver, and presumably this accounts for most of the 'other' cholesterol returning to the liver.

In summary, the cholesterol absorbed in the intestine from both endogenous and dietary sources is transported out of the intestine in chylomicrons and makes its way to the liver in the chylomicron remnants via chylomicron receptors (apoE and perhaps intestinal apoB receptors). During passage from the gut to the liver, chylomicrons may receive some free cholesterol from tissues and some cholesterol esters from other lipoproteins via cholesterol transport protein. VLDL secreted from the liver contains some cholesterol. During its catabolism it is largely catabolized to LDL. Some of the LDL is catabolized by peripheral tissues and some by the liver. VLDL and LDL can receive cholesterol esters from HDL via cholesterol transport proteins. Thus, some of the LDL cholesterol returning from the liver comes from tissue sources. LDL is removed by the LDL (B/E receptor) and the control of this receptor depends upon the liver cholesterol content and may be sensitive to such things as the state of the enterohepatic circulation, i.e. more receptors when bile acid synthesis is high and less receptors when bile acids are returning in high concentrations to the liver. Further apoE containing lipoproteins may also be taken up by the LDL (apoB/E) or apoE receptors in the liver, providing another route for return of cholesterol to the liver.

While the overall scheme presented here is essentially correct, the specific control of the different processes and the absolute uptake and secretion rates of the liver need to be established for a variety of physiological variations and pathological deviations.

Hofmann: Some workers have proposed that diminishing cholesterol absorption by the administration of beta-sitosterol might enhance the efficacy of gallstone dissolution agents. What do you think?

Small: How beta-sitosterol diminishes cholesterol absorption is not clear. One possibility is that it inhibits the LCAT mechanism in the enterocyte. It seems that cholesterol absorption is very closely related to the activity of the LCAT enzyme in the intestine, so that if the LCAT enzyme is blocked, cholesterol absorption is decreased.

Dowling: Is there any specificity in the effect that bile acids have on the LDL receptor in the liver? Since chenodeoxycholic acid seems to increase the level of LDL in plasma and ursodeoxycholic acid does not, one wonders if these two bile acids have different effects on the LDL receptor.

Small: The situation is not clear at present. What has been done is the following. Bile acid synthesis has been induced in dogs by cholestyramine administration. This is known to induce the LDL receptor. Then taurocholate was infused, and it was found that surface activity of the LDL receptor fell to extremely low levels in 5 h. Thus, in these experiments, taurocholate infusion lowered the level of LDL receptors which had been previously increased by cholestyramine administration. No other bile salts have been used to date in such studies. This work is difficult to interpret because the $T_{1/2}$ of the receptor in these studies − about 2 or 3 h − is much faster than the $T_{1/2}$ for the LDL receptor in tissue culture, when it is much longer. Indeed, *in vitro* the effect of cholesterol or bile acids on the LDL receptor requires at least 10−12 h of a stimulus before a change in LDL receptor activity is observed. So if this effect of bile salt is real, it seems unlikely to be an influence on the receptor synthesis, but rather some kind of physicochemical interaction, such as an 'internalization'. Obviously, there is much more to be done along this line.

La Russo: Dr Small, you said that the state of the enterohepatic circulation and hormones did not have an important effect on the level of the E receptor in the hepatocyte. What does influence the activity of the E receptor?

Small: The E receptor seems very hard to saturate. It takes up chylomicron remnants with an extraordinary avidity and oestrogen does not seem to influence its activity. There is no effect of interruption of the enterohepatic circulation. The LDL receptor behaves quite differently. It is stimulated by cholestyramine, oestrogen in the rat, thyroid hormones, etc.

Carey: When HDL is taken up by the liver, does it down-regulate the apoE receptor?

106

Small: Things are really more complicated than I implied, but I did not discuss the matter fully. The LDL receptor is considered to be rather non-specific, in that it mediates the uptake of both particles containing both apoA and apoE. Indeed, to measure apoE one must do it by difference. In practice, one exposes the system to particles containing apoB or apoB and E, and then obtains the apoE activity by difference. If one has molecules containing E apoprotein and cholesterol, one down-regulates the LDL receptor because of the LDL pathway. But this does not seem to influence the E receptor which is not down-regulated by the cholesterol in the liver. The liver can be full of cholesterol but the chylomicron receptor keeps right on working.

Carey: What flux of taurocholate was used in the experiment you described?

Small: The doses of taurocholate used were quite high, simulating what one might expect to come back to the liver after contraction of the gallbladder.

Erlinger: Does anyone know what is the influence of a conventional serum cholesterol-lowering agent, such as clofibrate, on the E receptor?

Small: I do not think this has been studied as yet. Indeed, the difference between the LDL and the apoE receptor was only discovered very recently. It seems very clear that there must be a receptor for chylomicrons because patients with familial homozygous hypercholesterolaemia, who have no B receptors in their body and whose liver will not take up LDL, clear chylomicrons absolutely normally. Such patients must have a receptor for the chylomicron remnant.

Von Bergman: Dr Small, I am confused about certain things. Is there a different receptor in the peripheral tissues? In the homozygote with familial cholesterolaemia, there does not seem to be any problem with total bile acid synthesis. Is the cholesterol which is synthesized to bile acids in patients with homozygous familial hypercholesterolaemia only due to the chylomicron remnant cholesterol which comes to the liver, or not?

Small: I think the cholesterol pools do exchange with each other. In patients with familial hypercholesterolaemia the liver does synthesize cholesterol. It can be returned to the liver by HDL whose uptake may involve the E receptor. When you eat eggs, you push the apoE up, and that seems to be a protective way of clearing your body of the extra cholesterol obtained in the diet. The only thing which the patient with familial homozygous cholesterolaemia cannot do is to take up low-density lipoproteins.

Dowling: There now follows another paper on a related topic. Lysosomes have been implicated in many diseases, and now we will hear about yet another contribution of lysosomes: Nick LaRusso is going to tell us about circulating lipoproteins, hepatic lysosomes and biliary lipids.

LaRusso: I would like to present some recent preliminary data which are consistent with the existence of a vesicular transport process in the hepatocyte that may be involved in the secretion of apolipoproteins and lipids into bile, perhaps via the processing of circulating lipoproteins in hepatic lysosomes.

Before I present these data I think it will be helpful to provide some background for those of you who are not familiar with the hepatocyte lysosome. Lysosomes are subcellular organelles which contain over 40 hydrolytic enzymes, all of which have an acid pH optimum (Fig. 5). These are prevented from entering the cytoplasm and damaging the cell because they are contained within a semipermeable, lipoprotein membrane. The major function of lysosomes is intracellular digestion. Recently, we and others have indicated that transport, storage and extracellular secretion of materials are also probably important lysosomal functions.

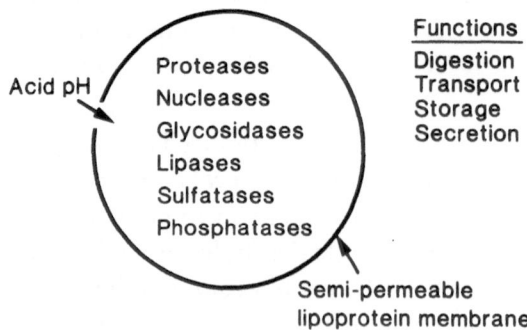

Figure 5 The lysosome

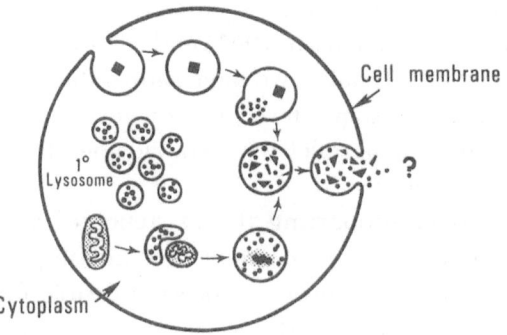

Figure 6   The lysosome-to-bile hepatic excretory pathway

Figure 6 depicts our present hypothesis concerning the lysosome-to-bile hepatic excretory pathway. Large molecular weight compounds can be incorporated into the hepatocyte by receptor-mediated or bulk-flow endocytosis, forming endocytic vesicles. These endocytic vesicles can then fuse with primary lysosomes, the lysosomes delivering hydrolytic enzymes which affect disassembly, disaggregation or digestion of the macromolecules. The vesicle is then known as a secondary lysosome. The fate of the disassembled macromolecule in the secondary lysosome depends in part on the molecular weight of the degradation products; small molecular weight digestive products may diffuse through the semipermeable lysosomal membrane to be reutilized by the cell; large molecular weight digestive products or molecules resistant to hydrolytic digestion remain sequestered within the secondary lysosome.

One possible fate for the secondary lysosome in the hepatocyte is fusion of the lysosomal membrane with the canalicular membrane and extrusion of the contents of the lysosome into bile. This process of 'cellular defaecation' by hepatocytes into bile was first suggested about 15 years ago.

We have accumulated a variety of biochemical data supporting the existence of this lysosome-to-bile hepatic excretory pathway. First, we have shown that there are lysosomal enzymes in bile, generally in quantities greater than enzymes from other cell organelles (LaRusso and Fowler, 1979). Second, we have demonstrated coordinate, or parallel, release of multiple lysosomal enzymes into bile, a finding consistent with bulk flow or exocytosis (LaRusso and Fowler, 1979). Third, we have shown alterations of the release of lysosomal enzymes into bile by microtubule binding agents (Sewell *et al.*, 1981) hormones (Lopez del Pino and LaRusso, 1981) and lysosomotropic compounds (Sewell *et al.*, 1982). Finally, we have shown that exogenous macromolecules which are sequestered in hepatocyte lysosomes are also secreted into bile in parallel with endogenous lysosomal enzymes (LaRusso *et al.*, 1982).

With these data supporting the existence of a lysosome-to-bile hepatic excretory pathway we began investigating the possible functions of this vesicular transport process. Possible functions include serving as a major route for the turnover of lysosomal constituents, involvement in biliary lipid and protein secretion, and regulation of biliary metal secretion. I would like to concentrate in this paper on the possible role of this pathway in the modulation of biliary lipid and protein secretion.

The hypothesis related to this aspect of our ongoing work is that the biliary excretion of lipids and apolipoproteins is modulated by the processing of circulating lipoproteins in hepatocyte lysosomes. The rationale for this hypothesis includes the following points. First, as was reviewed by Dr Small in the previous paper, lipoproteins are taken up by the liver and are sequestered in the hepatocyte lysosomes. Second, as I have just reviewed, hepatocyte lysosomes can release their contents directly into bile. Finally, other workers have suggested that biliary cholesterol and phospholipid are derived from a preformed pool of non-newly synthesized lipid, perhaps lipoproteins.

The aim of the study which I want to review in this paper was to determine if the protein and lipid components of lipoproteins can be excreted into bile after processing in hepatocyte lysosomes. This work was done in my laboratory in conjunction with Simon Mao, John Thistle, Richard Sewell and Toshio Kawamoto. The work is ongoing.

Our first experiment was simply to look for the presence of apolipoproteins in human bile. We then asked the question whether the apolipoproteins present in bile (see below) were derived from circulating lipoproteins and transported across the hepatocyte. We used the isolated perfused rat liver as our experimental model and examined bile before and after the addition of human lipoproteins to lipoprotein-free solutions perfusing isolated livers. We measured lipids by enzymatic methods, lysosomal enzymes by fluorometric assay, and apolipoproteins by radioimmunoassays specific for human apolipoproteins.

We examined human gallbladder bile obtained at surgery for the presence of apolipoproteins. We found apolipoproteins A-I, A-II, C-II and C-III in all the samples tested, in concentrations in the microgram range; we found no differences in the levels of apolipoproteins in bile from patients with and without gallstones (Sewell *et al.*, 1981).

Our results with the isolated perfused rat liver showed that apolipoproteins A-I and A-II, the major apolipoproteins of high-density lipoproteins (HDL), were present in bile after, but not before, addition of HDL to the lipoprotein-free perfusate (Kawamoto *et al.*, 1983).

We did an additional experiment in which we looked for the presence of apolipoprotein B, the major apolipoproteins of low-density lipoproteins (LDL) in the bile of isolated perfused rat livers from rats pretreated with ethinyl oestradiol, a hormone known to increase the uptake of LDL by the hepatocyte. Our results showed that apolipoprotein B was present in the bile of only those rats who had been treated with ethinyl oestradiol (Kawamoto *et al.*, 1983). In addition, the amount of cholesterol secreted into bile after addition of LDL to the perfusate was also increased in the rats given the hormone.

In summary, we have demonstrated that immunoreactive apolipoproteins are present in human bile, and that the apolipoprotein components of HDL and LDL, and perhaps the lipid components of LDL, can be transported across the liver and excreted into bile. We conclude from these data that the lysosome-to-bile hepatic excretory pathway may be involved in the biliary excretion of the lipid and protein components of lipoproteins.

Small: That is very exciting. I should tell you that when Dan Steinberg injected his sucrose-labelled LDL with radioactive sucrose, he showed that it went to the liver. He also found counts in the intestine and in the bile; I think about 15% of the total uptake by the liver actually ended up in the bile as sucrose. His data also suggest that part of the lipoprotein gets into bile. What bothers me a little bit is that the massive amounts of work on uptake of LDL show that the radioactive LDL molecule is broken down to rather small, sometimes non-TCA, precipitable material and that its immunoreactivity is lost. I wonder how you account for, presumably, whole molecules coming out in bile if you are assuming that they go through a pathway involving lysosomal fusion and digestion and exocytosis into bile.

LaRusso: I think that is a good question, Don. Let me say that we have no data on the physical form of the apolipoproteins in bile. We believe that the apolipoproteins in bile probably are present largely as intact polypeptides for two reasons. First, we see complete lines of identity between bile and antisera specific for human apolipoproteins in double immunodiffusion experiments, suggesting that the apolipoproteins in bile are at least of sufficient integrity to react with the antisera. Second, the amount of antibody needed to detect the levels of apolipoproteins measured in bile would also be consistent with a largely intact polypeptide. But you are absolutely right; if the lipoproteins go through the lysosome pathway, one would predict that there would be some breakdown. However, we do not know that for a fact, and it needs to be explored.

Carey: Is your isolated perfused rat liver dying all the time?

LaRusso: Not in our lab.

Carey: What do you use as a perfusate?

LaRusso: We use an oxygenation system consisting of silastic tubing which is permeable to oxygen. We perfuse the liver with Fluosol, which is a haemoglobin-free oxygen-carrying . . .

Carey: . . . it is in fact a detergent. That is why I asked the question, because the big point is whether it is in fact the equivalent of SDS with fluorine on it?

LaRusso: You asked the question, but you implied an answer with regard to the viability of the liver; I was just getting to that. The liver is variable by a variety of standard criteria; that is, oxygen uptake, LDH release into the perfusion medium, and bile flow. For $2\frac{1}{2}$–3 h, the liver works fine, as far as we can tell.

Carey: What of tight junctions and things like that?

LaRusso: I do not have any information on that, although a recent unpublished paper which I heard at the Midwest Gut Club compared the isolated rat liver perfused with Fluosol and with a haemoglobin-containing solution; there were no major differences.

Dowling: We must not get lost in the minutiae of the experimental design; perhaps you can discuss that afterwards.

Hofmann: I am not sure I understand your argument. But if I do understand your argument, the lipoproteins have something to do with biliary lipids.

LaRusso: That is one implication of these data, and I hope you are going to ask me what they might do?

Hofmann: I will if you want me to, but that was not my question. The question is this: if you perfuse your liver with a system that does or does not have lipoproteins and then add bile acids to introduce lecithin and cholesterol secretion, does the presence of lipoproteins make any difference?

LaRusso: In our system we have a constant infusion of taurocholate to help maintain bile flow, so we had not specifically looked at the variable. Certainly, that is one of the things that I am going to do when I get back, based on what I have learned about Bo Angelins' work. Does that answer your question?

Dowling: Just before we leave your presentation, as I understand it, you have been talking about a lysosomal shuttle taking apoproteins from blood and putting them into bile. Do they have an intracellular shuttle service to take new synthesized lipids and transport them to the canalicular membrane?

LaRusso: Well, there was a part of the illustration (Fig. 6) which I did not address, which is the autophagic route; that is, lysosomes are the major organelles involved in basal protein catabolism. So, organelles such as mitochondria, endoplasmic reticulum, etc., are taken up into lysosomes by an unclear mechanism and degraded, both in terms of their protein and presumably their lipid components. Whether that autophagic route also releases some of its material into bile is unclear at this point.

Dowling: I was not talking so much about the degradation pathway as much as the transport of newly synthesized material from the microsomes, to replace lipid in canalicular membrane.

LaRusso: I think that is unlikely based on our present understanding of the major fractions of the lysosomes.

Dowling: We are going to pass on to the next section and discuss hepatic bile acid transport in further detail. Alan Hofmann has been working with his colleague, Dr Eamonn O'Maille on the structural requirements for bile acid transport.

Hofmann: The basic aims and experimental design that form my presentation are quite simple. First, a word of background. If one studies the dissolution of model gallstone *in vitro*, it is well known that such dissolution is quite slow. When one adds lecithin, which increases the equilibrium solubility of cholesterol, the rate of instantaneous dissolution actually decreases due to an 'interfacial barrier'. The current view is that model bile, i.e. a micellar solution of bile acid–lecithin with or without cholesterol, contains both simple micelles composed of just bile acid molecules or predominantly bile acid molecules and mixed micelles containing bile acid and lecithin. The kinetic data obtained in the laboratory of Higuchi *et al.* (1973) suggests that the simple micelle mediates the transfer of cholesterol from the crystal to the mixed micelle. It is believed that the surface of the cholesterol crystal becomes negatively charged because of the adsorption of bile acid molecules, and that there is electrostatic repulsion between the negative surface of the crystal and the negatively charged simple micelle. If this hypothesis is correct, neutralization of either the charge on the crystal surface or the charge on the mixed micelle should accelerate the dissolution rate. The micelle can be neutralized by the addition of a cationic amphipathic molecule, such as cetyl trimethylammonium bromide, and when such cationic amphipathic agents are added the dissolution rate is accelerated greatly. We all agree that it would be desirable to be able to induce rapid gallstone dissolution in patients.

For some years we have thought that it would be desirable to find a cationic amphipathic compound which would be secreted in high concentrations into bile and thus accelerate gallstone dissolution. The obvious candidate molecules to try would be bile acids with a positive charge. Accordingly, in collaborative experiments with Dr M. Sawkat Anwer and Dr E. R. L. O'Maille, a visiting scholar from the University of Liverpool, we explored the effect of side-chain charge on bile acid uptake and transport using both acute bile fistula animals, as well as the isolated perfused liver.

The kinds of compounds we used and their pK_a values are shown here. The steroid nucleus was always cholic acid. We synthesized a di-anionic conjugate, cholyl aspartate. We used taurocholate as the mono-anionic compound. We also synthesized cholyl cysteate, which also has two charges. We obtained a zwitterionic bile acid having a minus and a plus charge, these having recently been synthesized by Larry Hjelmeland. We had three cationic bile acids available to us. We had two weakly basic compounds, cholylglycyl histamine and the primary amine cholylamine. These are partially ionized at physiological pH. Finally, we had cholylamine, which is iso-steric with cholyltaurine, except the sulphonic acid has been replaced by a quaternary ammonium group, so that the compound is fully positively charged at any pH value.

When we injected these compounds into animals we discovered that cholylamine was fully cholestatic. In further studies we found that there was modest entry of the uncharged cationic bile acids into the liver cell, but no excretion in bile for any of the compounds, except the mono-anionic and di-anionic compounds. Thus, in summary, it seems that mono-anionic bile acids can enter the liver cell well, and are highly concentrated into bile. Compounds which are partially uncharged at physiological pH, such as weakly acidic or weakly basic bile acids, can probably enter the liver cell passively. Only anionic compounds are secreted into bile. Zwitterionic and fully cationic compounds do not enter the liver cell at all. Di-anionic bile acids enter the liver cell poorly but are well excreted into bile.

Carey: Is not this information rather similar to the work of Leon Lack on ileal transport of bile acids?

Hofmann: Yes, it is; and we were inspired by his excellent structure–activity work. Obviously we had more interest in getting a cationic compound across than Lack did. I have no disagreement whatsoever with his work, which I think is of outstanding quality. My view is that bile acid transport into bile involves two sequential steps, and these may have different charge requirements. I might note that all structure–activity relationships are complex and one never changes one thing at once.

Carey: What is the Krafft point of cholylglycyl histamine?

Hofmann: I do not know, but it is below room temperature. The compound is quite water-soluble, but comes out of solution about pH 8 because the free base is not soluble. With respect to pH, its solubility is exactly opposite to that of an ordinary bile acid. It is soluble at acid pH, and not at alkaline pH.

Paumgartner: Do you have any data on the actual transport maximum of cholylglycyl histamine? Some years ago we examined the behaviour of tracer amounts of iodinated cholylglycyl histamine and found it behaved quite similarly to ^{14}C-labelled taurocholate in dogs. Do you have any information on the transport maximum of this cationic bile acid?

Hofmann: I think it is quite low, because we never got appreciable concentrations into bile.

Balistrieri: What is the sodium dependency for transport of these various compounds?

Hofmann: We have not studied it. I would assume that there must be a sodium dependency for any anionic compound. One of the reasons to study the zwitterionic compound was to see if we could find a compound which did not have a sodium dependency; but as you can see, it really does not enter the liver cell at all.

Dowling: Serge Erlinger is going to discuss another aspect of side-chain structure and bile acid transport.

Erlinger: This is an even more simple study than Hofmann's, and I will completely agree with him that there are at least two steps in bile acid transport by the liver, the uptake step and the secretion step.

It has been widely assumed, mostly on the basis of previous studies from our laboratory and others, that the secretion step was limiting in the overall transport process by the liver. Mostly because the maximal capacity for uptake is far in excess of the so-called maximal capacity for secretion. But one sometimes forgets that when one gives an unconjugated bile acid, there is a conjugation in between. And we asked the question, is conjugation important for secretion using non-toxic bile acid which is ursodeoxycholate and its tauro-conjugate, tauroursodeoxycholate.

116

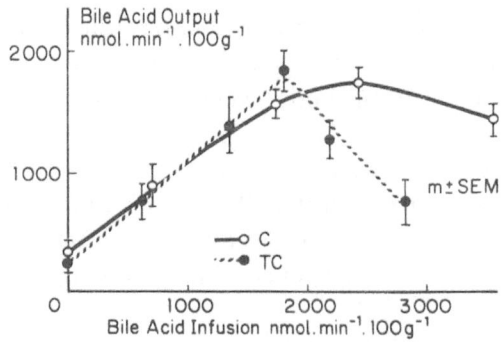

Figure 7

First I want to show what happens when one does the experiment with cholate and taurocholate (Fig. 7). This is the relationship between bile acid output and bile acid infusion when one gives cholate and its tauroconjugate (Fig. 7). You can see that output increases when infusion rate increases, up to a maximal value which we should call, perhaps, the maximal secretory rate, and after that output decreases. You can see that there is no apparent difference between the maximal output of cholate and that of taurocholate. This is probably because after this maximal value has been reached there is a decreased output, presumably due to toxicity of both the compounds. This is why we used urso (which is much less toxic) to see whether conjugation had an importance.

When one gives urso and one increases the infusion rate, the output increases up to a maximal value which is in the range of 800 nmol min^{-1} (100 g body weight)$^{-1}$ (Fig. 8).

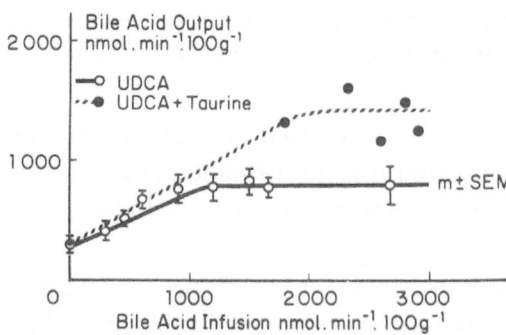

Figure 8

117

As mentioned previously when one does this type of experiment there is taurine depletion so at the same time we gave taurine. We were able to increase this maximal secretion rate up to about 1600 nmol min^{-1} 100 g body weight^{-1}. So that is the maximal capacity of secretion for urso.

When one gives tauro–urso one can see that the maximal secretion rate is much higher than that of unconjugated urso, which was low there and it is about 8 times higher with tauro–urso than it was with urso, even in the presence of taurine (Fig. 9).

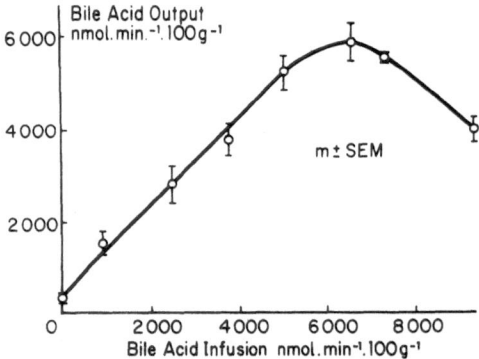

Figure 9

I think that we can reasonably conclude that at least for certain acids, such as urso, conjugation is the limiting step in the overall transport from plasma into bile. The reason why this is so is unclear, but it may be related to the low solubility of this bile acid in water.

Okolicsani: I am wondering if your rats were under general anaesthesia. Recent work suggested that general anaesthesia lowers the excretory capacity of other anionic ions, such as bilirubin. Do you think that this is an important variable in your experiments?

Erlinger: All studies were carried out under general anaesthesia, so that any effect on anion transport should apply equally to unconjugated ursodeoxycholate and tauroursodeoxycholate.

Okolicsani: Yes, but in rats it is well known that taurocholate increases the maximal biliary excretion of bilirubin, and this effect might have a bearing on your results.

Erlinger: I agree with the observation you cite, but that is not the point of my presentation.

Von Bergmann: I have two questions. First, $6000\ \text{ng min}^{-1}$ ($100\ \text{g body weight})^{-1}$ was approximately the maximum you infused. That is $200-300\ \text{mg}$, or $50\ \mu\text{mol/min}$, which is really a huge dose. Are you not worried about toxic effects of haemolysis?

Erlinger: There is no haemolysis with tauroursodeoxycholate.

Von Bergmann: You are aware of an old abstract from Hardison who showed that the apparent secretory T_m of bile acids was actually influenced by the diameter of the cannula used for bile duct cannulation. Is this an important variable in your experiment?

Erlinger: We are certain that this is not important. We used a large cannula.

Hofmann: You must admit that the dog is very special. If we infuse unconjugated bile acids into a hamster to the point of taurine depletion, he will immediately switch over and conjugate with glycine. So the dog is a special species. We may have to say that the conjugation is rate-limiting for certain species which, in presence of taurine depletion, cannot conjugate with glycine.

Erlinger: It may be so. There may be species differences.

Fromm: Can such concentrations be reached if the bile acids are infused intestinally.

Erlinger: I think this is an important question. I would assume that if you give physiological concentrations in the intestine, that the liver should be able to conjugate them.

Dowling: Dr Sauerbruch will now discuss the effects of sphincterotomy with and without cholecystectomy on bile acid and biliary lipid metabolism.

Sauerbruch: It has been pointed out in this symposium in several discussions that the sphincter of Oddi may have an important role in regulation of the enterohepatic cycling of bile acids. Although endoscopic sphincterotomy has become a widely used procedure for removal of some bile duct stones, it is still unknown to what extent this procedure might influence the enterohepatic circulation of bile acids and thus have a secondary effect on biliary lipid composition.

We therefore determined total bile acid pool size by isotope dilution and lipid content of hepatic bile in three patients with intact gall-bladders and three patients without gallbladders shortly after endo-scopic sphincterotomy, as well as 6–9 months after endoscopic sphincterotomy. Bile was obtained by direct cannulation of the common bile duct.

What we observed was that shortly after endoscopic sphincter-otomy the total bile acid pool size in the patients with intact gall-bladders ranged between 80 and 110 μmol/kg. In cholecystectomized patients who had sphincterotomy, the exchangeable bile acid pool was much lower, ranging between 35 and 50 μmol/kg.

In the patients with intact gallbladders the total bile acid pool size decreased in all patients to values between 15 and 50 μmol/kg 6–9 months later. This decrease was much more pronounced in the patients with intact gallbladders, suggesting that the effect of sphincterotomy on bile acid pool size was unrelated to the presence of the gallbladder.

Although the total bile acid pool size decreased in all patients, there were only minor changes in the molar percentages of individual bile acids, and the same was true for cholesterol and phospholipid.

The total lipid content increased in all patients, and this increase in total lipid content, together with minor changes in the mole percentages of individual biliary lipids, led to a slight decrease in the saturation index in four patients and a slight increase in two patients. The saturation index was calculated according to Cary and Small.

These data suggest that the sphincter of Oddi does have an important role in regulation of the size of the bile acid pool. The data further suggest that a reduction in the total bile acid pool may occur and need not necessarily increase the lithogenicity of hepatic bile. Our observations certainly could be explained by a marked enhancement of the enterohepatic cycling frequency of the bile acid pool after sphincterotomy.

Small: When Shaffer and Small (1977) measured secretion rates and pool size in patients with and without gallstones, or before and after cholecystectomy, he plotted the secretion rate versus the pool size. For those patients who had no gallbladders the extrapolation went through zero, indicating that all of the bile acid pool was involved in the enterohepatic circulation. When he plotted the data from the four patients who had gallbladders, another line was obtained which was parallel to the first line, but intercepted the ordinate above zero, indicating that there appeared to be part of the exchangeable pool which did not circulate. I wonder what happens if you treat patients with gallstones by sphincterotomy alone.

Sauerbruch: We have only measured hepatic bile in our studies, so we do not know what happens to gallbladder bile after sphincterotomy in the presence of an intact gallbladder. In addition, I think we have studied too few patients to be certain that the saturation index actually is lowered by sphincterotomy.

Hofmann: A recent abstract from Van Trappen suggests that if one measures the pool size by the Grundy technique in which one determines the specific activity of bile acid during continuous cycling of the pool, a falsely low value is obtained because not all of the pool circulates. How did you measure the pool size in your patients?

Sauerbruch: We measured the pool size by the intubation technique of Duane and collected bile by intubation.

Hofmann: It would seem to me that there is a risk in doing this procedure, because the technique of Duane *et al.* – the so-called one-shot pool size – has only been validated in patients who have an intact sphincter. Did you measure the pool size immediately after sphincterotomy to see if there was evidence of thorough mixing of the injected tracer?

Sauerbruch: Yes, we measured the pool size in patients before sphincterotomy using cholecystokinin to obtain gallbladder contraction. The coefficient variation of our measurements was about 5%.

Hofmann: That means your method is precise, but not necessarily accurate.

Carey: I would like to make a comment on the index of saturation. I know you corrected for total lipids and obtained a saturation percentage of 400–500. I think this is very interesting because quite recently we have shown that the actual metastability of dilute bile is enormous. The supersaturation observed in your samples is because the bile is extremely dilute, i.e. contains about 1–3% solids.

Dowling: Now a paper from the Bologna group by Dr Mazzella, who is going to tell us what happens to serum bile acids after pancreatico-biliary bypass.

Mazzella: Several kinds of biliopancreatic bypass (Scopinaro *et al.*, 1969) have been proposed in obese subjects to avoid the mixing of chyme with pancreatic and biliary secretion and to induce a selective malabsorption of fats. We studied conjugated cholic acid (CCA) and conjugated chenodeoxycholic acid (CCDCA) (by RIA) serum levels and faecal bile acid (BA) outputs (by gas-chromatographic method) in order to evaluate BA metabolism in three patients with biliopan-creatic bypass (BPB) and in six patients with biliopancreatic–jejunal bypass III (BPJP III). In BPB the contact of food with jejunum mucosa is preserved, but this does not happen in BPJP III.

The curve behaviour of serum bile acid levels obtained in BPB patients during 180 min was similar to behaviour details obtained in seven obese controls without surgical treatment: in fact both CCA and CCDCA peaked after meal. The behaviour observed in three BPJB III patients was completely different from that of control obese subjects and of BPB patients, since both CCA and CCDCA serum levels decreased after a meal.

Bile acid malabsorption was excluded when measuring bile acid outputs in BPJB III (420 ± 260 mg/day, mean $\pm$ SD) after 3-day stool collections which were found to be similar to those of obese controls (450 ± 300 mg/day, mean $\pm$ SD). In addition faecal bile acid pattern was also similar in the same groups.

A new protocol of study was performed: the area under curve (AUC) of CCA and CCDCA was evaluated both in response to a solid meal and to an infusion of cerulein ($2 \mu g/kg$) during 180 min in three other BPJB III patients. During the same period of time gallbladder motility was also monitored by HIDA. In two patients no emptying of gallbladder was evaluated after the meal, but it reached 75% after cerulein. In the third patient gallbladder could not be visualized at HIDA, as it was not functioning because of gallstones. Mean CCA and CCDCA AUCs after a meal were respectively: 0.10 (mean value $\mu mol/l \times 180$ min) and 0.285; after cerulein 0.80 and 1.63.

122

We may conclude that hormonal events might be responsible for the phenomena we observed, rather than bile acid malabsorption.

Dowling: We will have now two brief presentations before we finish. First, Dr Northfield will discuss briefly his studies on small bowel transit rate in patients with gallstones.

Northfield: I am going to present briefly a collaborative study carried out with my colleagues Drs Kupfer, Jazrawi and Maudgal, outlining our concept of the pathophysiology of the enterohepatic circulation of bile acids in cholesterol gallstone disease.

Dr Kupfer has studied small intestinal transit rate by the hydrogen breath test using a solid meal (Fig. 10). Transit time was significantly shorter in the gallstone patients (mean $\pm$ SEM 174 ± 10 min) than in the controls (223 ± 17 min; $p < 0.01$).

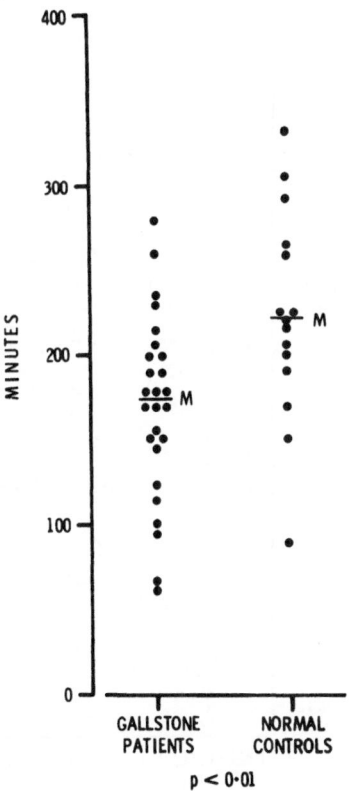

Figure 10   Small intestinal transport time

Dr Maudgal has previously shown that gallbladder emptying in response to a standard meal, expressed as a percentage decrease in gallbladder volume assessed by carefully standardized oral chole-cystogram, is gr ater for gallstone patients than for controls (46% vs 33%; $p < 0.01$). We have also demonstrated increased gallbladder sensitivity to CCK in gallstone patients indicated by a lower CCK threshold infusion rate to elicit a minimal detectable gallbladder contraction using radioisotope scanning ($p = 0.012$; Fig. 11). I would just like to point out that our methodology was somewhat different from that previously reported by Dr Forjacs in this meeting. Ours was a dose–response study using CCK, and it was the degree of gall-bladder emptying, not the rate, that we measured using a standard meal.

I would also like to remind you of the related data which Dr Jazrawi reported previously to this meeting – he studied six obese volunteers in hospital for 6 weeks, taking 600 calories daily. During half this time

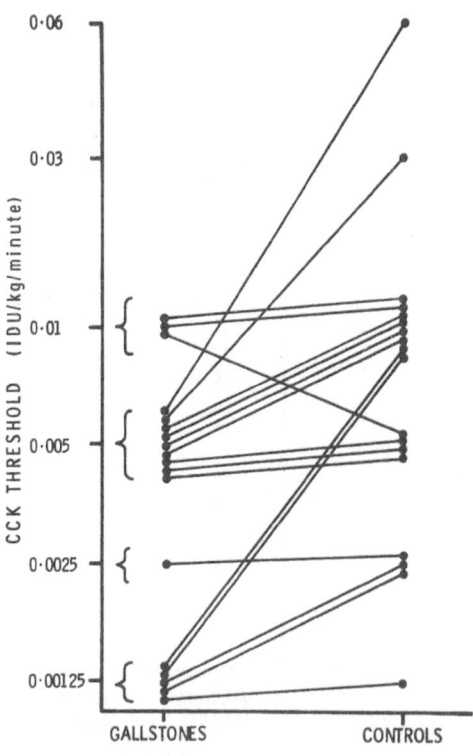

Figure 11 Gallbladder sensitivity to CCK in gallstone patients and controls

(random order) they received an intramuscular injection of 5 μg CCK octapeptide with each meal. During CCK, mean gallbladder emptying measured by isotope scanning rose from 50 to 78% ($p < 0.01$) and small intestinal transit time fell from 197 to 175 min (NS). Total bile acid pool size (Lindstedt technique) fell from 3.9 to 2.6 mM ($p < 0.01$; Fig. 12). Fractional turnover rate for [^{14}C]chenodeoxycholic acid rose from 0.20 to 0.38 per day ($p < 0.05$), providing indirect evidence of increased recycling frequency, but synthesis rate was unchanged, indicating a new steady state. Cholesterol saturation index (SI) of gallbladder bile rose from 1.4 to 1.8 ($p < 0.01$; Fig. 13). Dr Jazrawi has also shown in a separate experiment that artificial depletion of the bile acid pool increases SI by decreasing bile acid mass in the gallbladder without an equivalent decrease in cholesterol mass.

Figure 14 summarizes our concept of the pathophysiology of the enterohepatic circulation of bile acids in cholesterol gallstone disease. We believe that increased gallbladder sensitivity to CCK causes increased gallbladder emptying in response to a standard meal; there is also increased small intestinal transit rate leading to increased

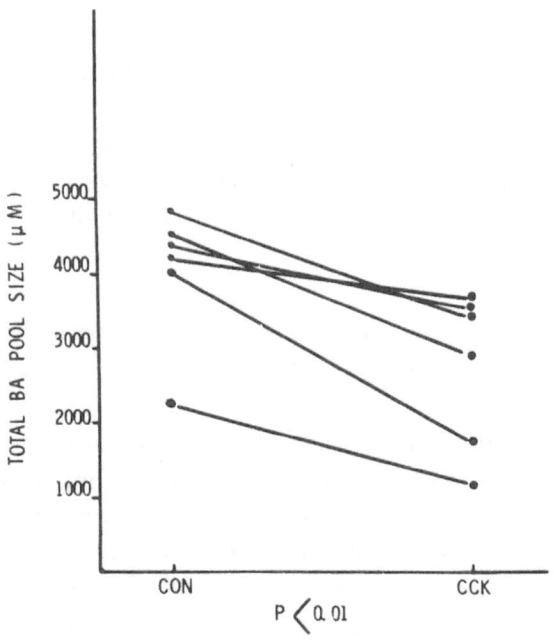

Figure 12　Total bile acid pool size, measured by the Lindstedt technique

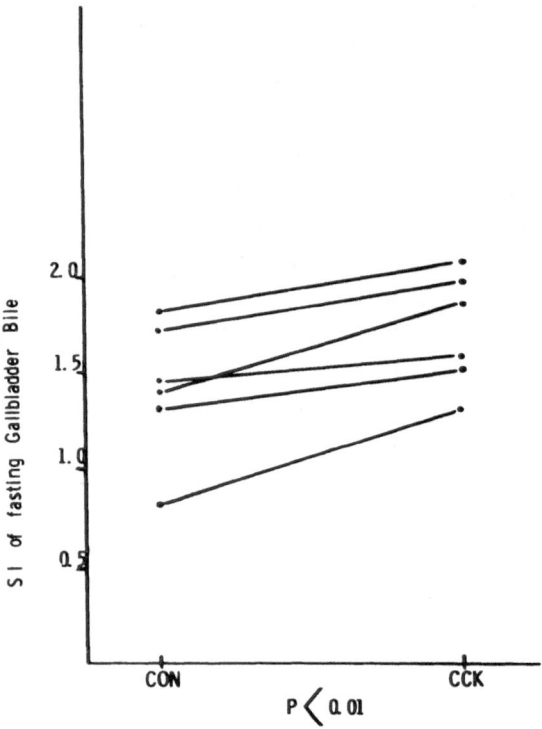

Figure 13   Cholesterol saturation index of gallbladder bile

recycling frequency of the pool. The increased recycling frequency leads to a reduced bile acid pool size, a reduction in bile acid mass in the gallbladder, and thus an increased SI of fasting gallbladder bile.

Dowling: Are there comments or questions or discussion? Dr Forjacs, you must want to offer a comment.

Forjacs: We also studied gallbladder contraction from the ultrasound data I showed, and I think that maybe the important thing is the actual movement of bile, and that is what we are looking at with HIDA, rather than gallbladder contraction, as I really discussed previously. One would not try to measure cardiac output, for example, by measuring the volume of the heart in systole and diastole, so perhaps the thing that we should be looking at is bile flow here.

126

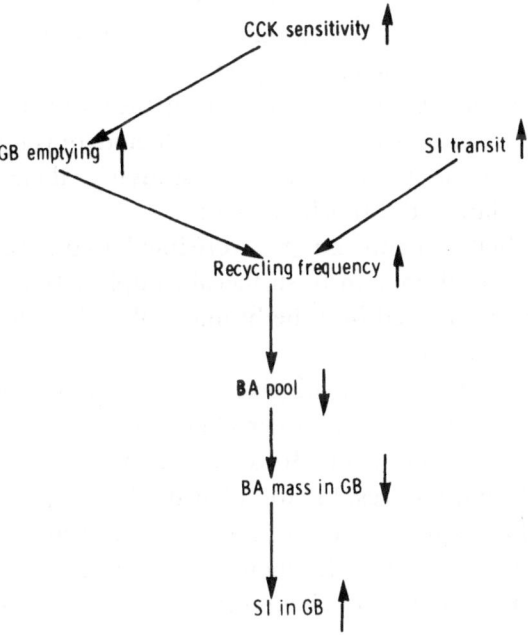

Figure 14 Pathophysiology of enterohepatic bile acid circulation in cholesterol gallstone disease

Northfield: I think that measuring the volume of the heart in systole and diastole might well give you stroke volume. I am just trying to emphasize that the methodology was different in our respective studies. I do not know if you want us to go on pursuing the differences in methodology.

Hofmann: Where does the hydrogen come from in the breath?

Northfield: This was with a solid meal, and baked beans was the main source of non-absorbable carbohydrate. The idea is that this results from exposure to the bacteria in the caecum, and we have validated in the gallstone subjects that it does correspond with arrival of radioisotope in the caecum.

Dowling: We will now pass on to the last communication, and this is based on work done by Dr Franco Bazzoli when he was working with Dr Fromm in Pittsburgh; Dr Fromm will tell us about it.

Fromm: Since we have so far only touched upon the hepatic and biliary part of the enterohepatic circulation, I think it is now appropriate to finally move into the enteral part.

The aim of the study was to gain further information on the comparative hepatotoxic potential of chenodeoxycholic (cheno) and ursodeoxycholic (urso) acids by studying their comparative 7-dehydroxylation to lithocholic acid.

Both labelled cheno and urso were incubated simultaneously under anaerobic conditions in fresh faecal samples. In addition, the compounds were infused into the human colon as well as into the colon of a rhesus monkey.

If the results of all 14 subjects studied were considered, there was no statistical difference between cheno and urso in their 7-dehydroxylation to lithocholic acid. However, when we looked at the individual biotransformation results we identified two populations. In one group, the majority of the subjects, the biotransformation to lithocholic acid was identical, whereas in the other there was a slightly faster transformation of cheno than of urso to lithocholic acid (Figs. 15 and 16).

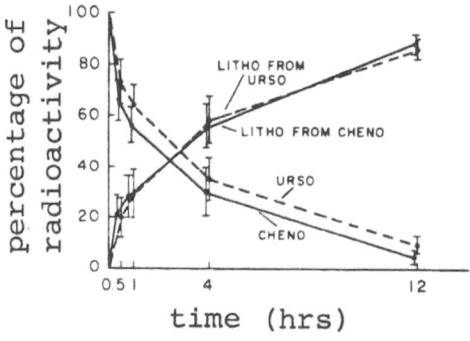

Figure 15 Formation of [^{14}C]lithocholic acid (litho) from [^{14}C]chenodeoxycholic acid (cheno) and [^{14}C]ursodeoxycholic acid (urso), *in vitro* in faecal anaerobic incubates in 10 subjects. In these cases the formation of litho from cheno was very similar to that from urso

The influence of different concentrations of precursors, cheno and urso, on the 7-dehydroxylation was also investigated. There was no significant change in the biotransformation pattern when the concentrations of the incubated precursors were increased or decreased.

The *in-vivo* biotransformation results after infusion of cheno and urso, respectively, into the human colon confirmed the *in-vitro*

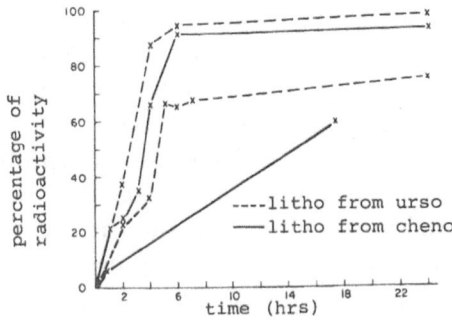

Figure 16 Formation of [^{14}C]lithocholic acid (litho) from [^{14}C]chenodeoxycholic acid (cheno) and [^{14}C]ursodeoxycholic acid (urso), *in vitro* in faecal anaerobic incubates in four subjects. In these cases cheno converted significantly faster than urso to litho at 1 and 4 h ($p < 0.05$)

studies. In fact, the 7-dehydroxylation of cheno and urso to lithocholic acid was comparable (Fig. 17). Similar observations were made when these compounds were infused into the colon of a rhesus monkey. Both in bile fistula and in the colon the amount of lithocholic acid formed from cheno was found to be similar to that formed from urso.

In summary, the 7-dehydroxylation of cheno and urso to lithocholic acid is very similar. However, there appears to be a sub-population in which the formation of lithocholic acid from cheno is somewhat faster than from urso. We interpret the results as follows: in most cases the risk of liver damage from lithocholic acid *formation* seems to be very similar for cheno and urso. However, there appears to be a sub-population of subjects in whom the risk of liver toxicity from lithocholic acid is higher from cheno than from urso.

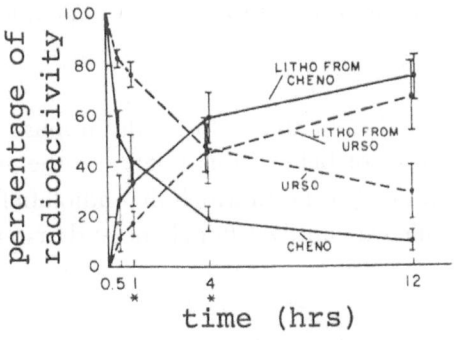

Figure 17 Formation of [^{14}C]lithocholic acid (litho) after colonic instillation of [^{14}C]ursodeoxycholic acid (urso) and [^{14}C]chenodeoxycholic acid (cheno) in four asymptomatic gallstone patients

Carey: I have heard you present these data before and there is a question that did not occur to me then that has occurred to me now. You have instilled *in-vivo* into the colon similar concentrations of urso and cheno, but once they arrive in the colon their physical state will change very quickly. Cheno will be soluble and probably get absorbed quickly. Urso may precipitate and crystals may bind to this and just undergo slow solution, giving off monomers over the whole length of the colon. In other words, the time that urso molecules are exposed to bacterial enzymes may be much longer than for the same concentration of cheno. Therefore conversion of urso was in fact slower. Normally you might have got the same speed because you had a much longer *in-vivo* incubation time.

Fromm: You are referring here to the *in-vivo* conditions. Theoretically speaking, there is, of course, a difference in the solubility between cheno and urso, but in the patients in whom we have infused these bile acids into the colon, the colonic pH was quite acid, and neither cheno nor urso would be solubilized. Furthermore, in the rhesus monkey, in which cheno and urso were instilled into the colon, the appearance of lithocholic acid was measured both in colonic samples and in bile fistula bile. Under these conditions the lithocholic acid formation was again found to be very similar for both epimers.

Hofmann: It seems to me that you cannot equate formation with absorption? It is quite possible that people taking cheno and urso, both converted to litho, but because the litho is solubilized better in cheno than in urso, that the input of litho into the enterohepatic circulation could be considerably greater in people taking cheno than urso?

Fromm: Again, I do not think this really applies to the colon. The reason that I do not believe this relates to the study in the rhesus monkey with a bile fistula, in which the radiolabelled lithocholic acid appearing in bile was similar after cheno and urso instillation into the colon.

Hofmann: I actually think we have to do litho kinetics in people taking urso and compare them to litho kinetics of people taking cheno until we have the final answer.

Fromm: I agree that such studies would be in order.

Paumgartner: I missed the number of patients you studied, but since you talked of a sub-population, I would be interested if you have a bi-modal distribution of the transformation rates of cheno to litho. You said it is a sub-population. Did you have a continuous distribution of these rates or was it bi-modal?

Fromm: We have conducted *in-vitro* biotransformation studies on faecal samples of 14 subjects. Repeated studies in the same subject did not show any changes in the biotransformation pattern.

Paumgartner: But in the population, do you have a bi-modal distribution of rate or a continuous distribution?

Fromm: The distribution was bi-modal rather than continuous. There were four patients in whom cheno was converted faster than urso to lithocholic acid, whereas in the remaining 10 subjects the litho formation from cheno and urso was almost identical.

REFERENCES

Albers, J. J., Grundy, S. M., Cleary, P. A., *et al.* (1982). The effect of chenodeoxycholic acid on lipoproteins and apolipoproteins. *Gastroenterology*, **82**, 638

Bennion, L. J. and Grundy, S. M. (1975). Effects of obesity and caloric intake on biliary lipid metabolism in man. *J. Clin. Invest.*, **56**, 996

Gilmore, I. T., Barnhart, J. L., Hofmann, A. F., *et al.* (1982). Effects of individual taurine-conjugated bile acids on biliary lipid secretion and sucrose clearance in the unanaesthetized dog. *Am. J. Physiol.*, **242**, G40

Goldstein L. J. and Brown, M. S. (1977). Atherosclerosis: the low density lipoprotein hypothesis. *Metabolism*, **26**, 1257

Higuchi, W. I., Prakonpan, S. and Young, F. (1973). Mechanisms of dissolution of human cholesterol gallstones. *J. Pharm. Sci.*, **62**, 945

Kawamoto, T., Kost, L. J., Sewell, R. B., *et al.* (1983). Biliary excretion of the protein and lipid components of lipoproteins. *Hepatology* (abstr; in press)

LaRusso, N. F. and Flower, S. (1979). Coordinate secretion of acid hydrolases in rat bile: Hepatocyte exocytosis of lysosomal protein? *J. Clin. Invest.*, **64**, 948

LaRusso, N. F., Kost, L. J., Carter, J. A., *et al.* (1982). Triton WR-1339, a lysosomotropic compound, is excreted into bile and alters the biliary excretion of lysosomal enzymes and lipids. *Hepatology*, **2**, 209

Lopez del Pino, V. and LaRusso, N. F. (1981). Dissociation of bile flow and biliary lipid secretion from biliary lysosomal enzyme output in experimental cholestasis. *J. Lipid Res.*, **22**, 229

Sama, C., LaRusso, N. F., Lopex del Pino, V., *et al.* (1982). Effects of acute bile acid administration on biliary lipid secretion in healthy volunteers. *Gastroenterology*, **82**, 515

Scopinaro, N., Gianetta, E., Civalleri, D., *et al.* (1979). Bilio-pancreatic by-pass for obesity. I. An experimental study in dogs. *Br. J. Surg.,* **66**, 613

Sewell, R. B., Kost, L. J., Carter, J. A., *et al.* (1981). Hormones and microtubular binding agents selectively alter biliary lysosomal protein secretion. *Gastroenterology,* **80**, 1281 (abstr.)

Sewell, R. B., Kost, L. J., Kawamoto, T., *et al.* (1982). Chloroquine alters the biliary excretion of lipids and lysosomal protein. *Gastroenterology,* **82**,1176 (abstr.)

Sewell, R. B., Mao, S. J. T. and LaRusso, N. F. Apolipoproteins are present in human bile. *Hepatology,* **1**, 545 (abstr.)

Shaffer, E. A. and Small, D. M. (1977). Biliary lipid secretion in cholesterol gallstone disease. *J. Clin. Invest.,* **59**, 828

Index